SKILLS TRAINING
IN PSYCHODYNAMIC PSYCHOTHERAPY

SKILLS TRAINING IN PSYCHODYNAMIC PSYCHOTHERAPY

A Problem-Focused Approach

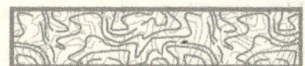

FREDRIC N. BUSCH

THE GUILFORD PRESS
New York   London

Copyright © 2026 The Guilford Press
A Division of Guilford Publications, Inc.
www.guilford.com

All rights reserved

Except as indicated, no part of this book may be reproduced, translated, stored in a retrieval system, or transmitted, in any form or by any means, electronic, mechanical, photocopying, microfilming, recording, or otherwise, without written permission from the publisher.

Printed in the United States of America

This book is printed on acid-free paper.

For product and safety concerns within the EU, please contact GPSR@taylorandfrancis.com, Taylor & Francis Verlag GmbH, Kaufingerstraße 24, 80331 München, Germany.

Last digit is print number: 9 8 7 6 5 4 3 2 1

LIMITED DUPLICATION LICENSE

These materials are intended for use only by qualified mental health professionals.

The publisher grants to individual purchasers of this book nonassignable permission to reproduce all materials for which photocopying permission is specifically granted in a footnote. This license is limited to you, the individual purchaser, for personal use or use with clients. This license does not grant the right to reproduce these materials for resale, redistribution, electronic display, or any other purposes (including but not limited to books, pamphlets, articles, video or audio recordings, blogs, file-sharing sites, internet or intranet sites, and handouts or slides for lectures, workshops, or webinars, whether or not a fee is charged). Permission to reproduce these materials for these and any other purposes must be obtained in writing from the Permissions Department of Guilford Publications.

This publication is intended to provide helpful and informative material. It is not intended to diagnose, treat, cure, or prevent any health problem or condition, nor is it intended to replace the advice of a health professional. No action should be taken based solely on the contents of this book. Always consult your physician or qualified health care professional on any matters regarding your health and before adopting any suggestions in this book or drawing inferences from it.

The author and publisher specifically disclaim all responsibility for any liability, loss, or risk, personal or otherwise, which is incurred as a consequence, directly or indirectly, from the use or application of any contents of this book.

Any and all product names referenced within this book are the trademarks of their respective owners. Always read all information provided by the manufacturers' product labels before using their products. The author and publisher are not responsible for claims made by manufacturers.

Library of Congress Cataloging-in-Publication Data is available from the publisher.

ISBN 978-1-4625-5885-8 (paper)
ISBN 978-1-4625-5891-9 (cloth)

To my family

About the Author

Fredric N. Busch, MD, is Clinical Professor of Psychiatry at Weill Cornell Medical College (WCMC) and a faculty member of the Columbia University Center for Psychoanalytic Training and Research (CPTR). His research and writing, including several books, have focused on topics including psychodynamic approaches to specific disorders, integrating psychotherapy and medication, and problem-focused psychodynamic psychotherapy. Dr. Busch was involved in developing panic-focused psychodynamic psychotherapy, the first psychodynamic treatment of a DSM anxiety disorder to demonstrate efficacy. He teaches and supervises problem-focused psychodynamic psychotherapy at WCMC and chairs courses in psychoanalytic research, combined treatment, and neuropsychoanalysis at CPTR. Dr. Busch is the recipient of teaching and research awards from the American Psychoanalytic Association, CPTR, and WCMC, and is a Distinguished Fellow of the American Psychiatric Association.

Contents

	Introduction	1
CHAPTER 1	Core Psychodynamic Concepts and Models	5
CHAPTER 2	Identifying Problems	23
CHAPTER 3	Identifying and Addressing the Situations, Emotions, Thoughts, and Developmental Factors Contributing to Problems	59
CHAPTER 4	Identifying and Addressing Self and Other Representations	85
CHAPTER 5	Addressing Intrapsychic Conflicts and Defenses	109
CHAPTER 6	Developing Mentalization Skills	133
CHAPTER 7	Clarifying the Psychodynamic Formulation and Using It as a Framework of Interventions	151

CHAPTER 8	Working Through	174
CHAPTER 9	Termination	193
	References	213
	Index	216

Purchasers of this book can download and print copies of the reproducible handouts and worksheets at *www.guilford.com/busch-forms* for personal use or use with clients (see copyright page for details).

Introduction

Psychoanalysts historically have avoided focusing on specific problems in therapy, believing that such an approach does not address the underlying structure of the "neurosis" and distorts the transference relationship, considered to be a core therapeutic tool. However, many analysts in recent years have viewed these concerns as misplaced and inaccurate and have developed a series of disorder and symptom focused manualized treatments (e.g., Bateman & Fonagy, 2016; Busch et al., 2016, 2021; Yeomans et al., 2015). Manualization enables systematic assessment of these treatments, and research studies have demonstrated their effectiveness (Clarkin et al., 2007; Milrod et al., 2007, 2016; Storebo et al., 2020). This book expands on a manualized treatment called problem-focused psychodynamic psychotherapy (PrFPP; Busch, 2022), a modified psychoanalytic approach that targets the identification, understanding, and amelioration of specific problems.

This book is designed to describe and demonstrate how a therapist uses PrFPP to address the set of problems (e.g., symptoms, relationship difficulties, behavioral issues) the patient presents with. To be clear, the focus in using PrFPP is on the constellation of problems the patient brings to therapy, rather than on a particular disorder. In PrFPP, the therapist works with the patient to develop a core psychodynamic formulation for problems, which is then used as a framework for targeted therapeutic interventions, and transference remains a significant tool of the treatment. The formulation and psychodynamic interventions will be familiar to psychoanalysts, but in PrFPP they are modified to target specific problems.

This text is meant to be of use to practicing psychodynamic clinicians, but it is also intended for training purposes for those less familiar with psychodynamic psychotherapy who wish to add techniques to their therapeutic armamentarium. The approaches are described in clear, user-friendly language that enables an understanding of what are sometimes presented as complex concepts.

The techniques described in this book include identifying specific problems to focus on and elaborating the context, thoughts, and emotions surrounding these problems, which also aid in developing self-observational capacities. Psychoeducation plays a greater part in this treatment than in traditional psychodynamic psychotherapies, as the therapist explains to the patient both the techniques of the treatment and how they are helpful. The therapist and patient together build a specific formulation for each problem, and that formulation is used as a framework for developing interventions. The components of the formulation include developmental contributors, self and other representations, intrapsychic conflicts and defenses, and mentalization disruptions. This psychodynamic treatment targets a reduction in problems, including a focus on behavioral change.

The use of worksheets provides an additional approach for identifying and addressing problems—including supporting patients as they apply new knowledge, insights, and psychodynamic skills outside of sessions, and after treatment terminates. Psychodynamic skills include:

1. The capacity to identify contexts and emotions likely to exacerbate problems and to employ interventions to address these triggers.
2. The capacity to identify and address the impact of the developmental history on problems.
3. The ability to identify and confront contributory negative self and other representations.
4. The ability to recognize and manage conflicted feelings and fantasies that exacerbate problems.
5. The use of mentalization skills to help address adverse perceptions of others that contribute to problems.
6. The employment of behavioral changes to better manage intrapsychic and interpersonal conflict.

These skills aid patients in the ultimate goal of therapy, gaining the capacity to manage their problems on their own. The worksheets used in PrFPP are valuable in helping patients to develop and practice these psychodynamic skills, leaving them with the ability to take steps themselves to contend with their problems.

HOW TO USE THE WORKSHEETS

The worksheets presented in this book are intended to aid in the therapeutic process of this treatment, to gain further information about contributors to a patient's problems, and to help patients to develop and practice psychodynamic skills. There are three ways of using the worksheets. One is as a guided interview, in which the therapist uses the worksheet questions to identify patients' specific problems and elaborate and address contributing factors. In this format, these questions are offered as a *guide*: Rather than follow them verbatim, the therapist can adjust them to follow the leads of the patient. In the second option, during a session the therapist and patient discuss the specific items detailed on a worksheet, and either the therapist or patient writes down the responses to the questions for further discussion. In a third option, the patient fills out the worksheets outside of sessions, and then the therapist and patient discuss the patient's responses in sessions.

As these worksheets are presented in the book, I occasionally make a suggestion as to which of the uses a worksheet works best. For instance, the evaluation of problems worksheets in Chapter 2 function best as guiding questions, whereas the worksheet in Chapter 3 to monitor problems and their triggers (Worksheet 3.1, p. 76) is most helpful for patients to fill out outside of sessions and bring in for discussion.

I realize that the use of such worksheets represents a significant departure from traditional notions of psychodynamic psychotherapy, and some therapists may find them inconsistent with their conception of this treatment approach. This psychotherapeutic approach can work effectively without using the worksheets clinically. Nevertheless, even if the worksheets are not given to patients, the questions on the worksheets can help therapists to plan and structure treatment, keeping the patient's problems in focus.

Over the course of my career, I have seen many patients who have been in prior psychodynamic treatments report that they gained an understanding of the forces that contributed to their feelings and behaviors but were *unable to make changes* in them. One source of this inability is that those prior treatments inadequately identified and addressed the multiple contributors to particular problems. I have found that the use of modified psychodynamic interventions that target specific problems, combined with the use of worksheets, aids in helping patients make changes and ease problems. Thus, this book equips therapists with techniques that help them to be more effective in their work with patients.

CHAPTER 1

Core Psychodynamic Concepts and Models

Psychodynamic psychotherapy continues to be the most widely used psychotherapeutic approach, but its reach and impact have been circumscribed due to limited systematic research, the continued use of complex terminology, and the tendency in the field to overvalue longer-term treatments to the detriment of shorter-term interventions. In writing this book, I hope to help make psychodynamic psychotherapeutic concepts and approaches more comprehensible and user friendly, shorter term, and therefore more accessible for clinical use in a world of larger caseloads and more limited health care resources. I do that largely through exploring practical ways of focusing psychodynamic approaches on patients' specific problems and describe interventions aimed at diminishing problems and their risk of recurrence, elaborating on a clinical approach called problem-focused psychodynamic psychotherapy (PrFPP; Busch, 2022). Such efforts include the development of a psychodynamic formulation or framework for specific problems that can enable more rapid and targeted psychodynamic interventions, addressing the needs of a broader range of patients, and creating more opportunities for systematic research. To further these goals, I have added worksheets to help patients process and apply treatment interventions.

To reach these goals, it is essential to use precise language and gain a shared understanding of what we mean by certain technical concepts in providing care for those suffering from mental disorders and psychological problems. Additionally, these concepts need to be communicated in clear, user-friendly language, both for mental health professionals to learn this treatment and to effectively communicate with patients. To that end, this chapter reviews core psychodynamic concepts that are used throughout the book in its description of problem-focused psychodynamic psychotherapy. These concepts are employed to elaborate a series of different psychodynamic theoretical models and associated clinical interventions. They are also used in describing the components of the psychodynamic formulation (Chapter 3), which provides a framework for interventions.

INTRAPSYCHIC FACTORS

The Role of the Unconscious in Symptoms and Problems

A core component of psychodynamic psychotherapy is that patients' symptoms/problems have meanings and contributors of which they are unaware, or **unconscious**. An essential technique in treatment is to make patients conscious of these factors, allowing for the development of interventions to relieve them. Patients may not be aware of some of these contributors (e.g., contexts that trigger symptoms, links to past experiences) simply because they have not attended to or considered them. Other factors, such as mental states and impulses that are experienced as emotionally dangerous or painful, are actively kept out of awareness, or repressed, becoming part of the **"dynamic unconscious"** (Freud, 1893–1895; Shapiro, 1992). However, repression is not totally effective, as these wishes press for expression. The potential emergence into consciousness of repressed wishes and feelings is experienced as threatening, unacceptable, or intolerable, triggering guilt and anxiety.

Internal struggles between wishes and fantasies and internalized prohibitions about them are referred to as **intrapsychic conflicts** (Freud, 1926). Certain wishes and feelings come to be seen as unacceptable as part of normal development and socialization by caregivers (and other environmental forces). Individuals from backgrounds with more severe traumatic or adverse events likely have a greater degree of conflict regarding sexual, aggressive, and attachment feelings and fantasies, as efforts to fulfill these wishes are experienced as more threatening. A sense of danger can develop from reactions of caregivers that are punitive, judgmental, or rejecting in response to such wishes as opposed to helping the child understand, modulate, and, if possible, express them in an appropriate manner (Bowlby, 1973). Over the course of development, fears and guilt surrounding these impulses are internalized, becoming experienced as a threat from the conscience or superego (Freud, 1926). Thus, the individual develops a judgment system that evaluates whether the particular wish or fantasy is safe, dangerous, or "bad" to acknowledge and express.

Two wishes can also be experienced as contradictory, such as to care for and to hurt another person, creating additional conflict, anxiety, and guilt. An important goal of psychoanalytic treatment is to bring these intrapsychic conflicts to conscious awareness. By making these wishes conscious, patients can consider the possibility that they are more tolerable and less dangerous than they believe. Additionally, the awareness enables patients to determine how to better manage or express these wishes.

Throughout this book, we describe how intrapsychic conflicts contribute to a variety of problems. Wishes to hurt or damage others, longings to be attached, and sexual fantasies are common sources of conflict. Aggressive fantasies of outdoing, harming, or dominating others can create conflict in various ways. For example, these wishes can cause fears of disrupting important attachment relationships and triggering retaliation. Although found in many problems or disorders, this dynamic is particularly common in anxiety, panic, and Cluster C personality disorders (Busch et al., 2012). Patients with such presenting problems often have a sense of fearful dependency on others that increases the perceived danger of angry fantasies, potentially causing a disruption in attachment. A sense of needing others becomes threatening when one believes others cannot be depended upon (that they will respond in hurtful and damaging ways), leaving one feeling unsafe in close attachment relationships. Because of the threat to dependency, individuals fear that angry feelings and fantasies may more readily disrupt these relationships.

Aggressive wishes toward others can also trigger guilt about harming others who are also loved. This conflict can lead to anger being turned inward in the form of self-criticism or self-punishment, a dynamic common in depressive disorders (Busch et al., 2016). Conflicted anger can be projected onto others (Abraham, 1911), who are then perceived as more attacking or rejecting than they may be in reality, intensifying anxiety, depression, and interpersonal problems.

Core wishes to be cared for (dependent) or intimate can trigger fears of rejection or intrusion and engulfment by others. These threats can feel particularly intense if the individual has experienced adverse developmental events or traumatic experiences that have increased the perceived danger of disrupting relationships, generating fears of being vulnerable with another person (Busch et al., 2021). Sexual wishes can trigger guilt and anxiety if they are experienced as difficult to control or inappropriate. Sexual desires may also combine with wishes for caretaking or aggressive fantasies, potentially leading to conflict about these sexual/dependent or sexual/aggressive fantasies.

This is not an exhaustive list; the therapist should attend to the particular nature of the emergence of patients' conflicts as they relate to specific problems. For example, patients with panic disorder often deny angry feelings toward people to whom they feel closely attached. An emerging conscious access to angry fantasies can trigger panic attacks and associated defenses (e.g., reaction formation and undoing; see below) that prevent any further awareness or enactment of the unacceptable wishes. The panic derives from the fear that any expression of anger would disrupt relationships, believed to be essential for security and safety (Busch et al., 1991; Shear et al., 1993). Psychodynamic treatment helps patients gain awareness of these angry fantasies and fears and the associated maladaptive patterns and symptoms. Panic diminishes as angry wishes and fantasies are verbalized and found to be less threatening than believed. Techniques for identifying and addressing such conflicts are addressed in Chapters 5 and 7.

CASE EXAMPLE: MR. A

Mr. A, a 48-year-old gay Latino writer and father of two, had long-standing anxiety and panic attacks that intensified late in the COVID-19 pandemic. During this time, he found that being in close quarters with his husband Joseph led Joseph to be more intrusive, putting pressure on Mr. A to structure his time more. For example, Joseph would come to his home office when he was working to press him to go outside, believing that Mr. A spending more time in the house would add to his anxiety. He felt unable to ask Joseph to step back for fear of making him angry. At the same time, Joseph had been increasingly busy at his career as an investment banker, while Mr. A's had slowed down. As the pandemic receded, this led to Joseph increasing travel for his work, triggering Mr. A's jealousy. He was aware of feeling relieved when his husband left on trips but also noted the continuation of anxiety and panic during Joseph's absence.

Mr. A described growing up in an environment in which there was little discussion of feelings. He was subjected to long harangues by his father about problems at his work and frustrations in his life. Although he and his sister felt both bored and marginalized by their father's preoccupations, the family had never developed the skills for expressing these feelings directly. His mother similarly yielded to his father's "lectures." At other times, his father would have temper episodes, attacking Mr. A and his sister, calling them "useless" or "entitled."

After he entered PrFPP, the therapist asked how Mr. A felt about the pressure from Joseph. Mr. A said he was aware of some frustration but struggled to feel it was okay or even express it. After all, his husband was just demonstrating concern about him, as he had tended to isolate and avoid his work during the pandemic. And he was worried about how Joseph might react to Mr. A expressing his frustration with their relationship. He was fearful that Joseph would lose his temper and insult him, despite such behavior being rare. However, as Mr. A felt safer in describing his feelings to the therapist, more intense irritation with his husband emerged, including thoughts about leaving him. The therapist formulated that he had never had an opportunity to express his anger growing up and even feared doing so based on his father's rages, leaving him with few skills to negotiate his needs with others. Feelings of anger felt dangerous and disruptive to him, creating conflict, and he would push them out of his mind (repress them). The therapist determined that it would be important to help Mr. A become aware of and feel safer with these feelings, and then consider how he might better address them with his husband.

Defense Mechanisms

Unacceptable or frightening fantasies and feelings are often kept from consciousness by psychological processes called **defense mechanisms** (A. Freud, 1936), of which the individual is typically unaware. In problem-focused psychodynamic psychotherapy, the therapist seeks to identify the presence and meanings of defenses. The therapist shares these with the patient, with the goal of revealing underlying painful or conflicted feelings and fantasies and associated defenses that contribute to problems and resolving the conflicts and intolerable emotions in a more adaptive way.

An example of a defense mechanism is **denial**, in which the individual disavows uncomfortable feelings or fantasies. An example of the use of denial is panic patients' lack of awareness of angry feelings and fantasies. For example, patients may deny ever feeling anger or do not acknowledge being irritated at others, even when anger would be an appropriate response to their behavior.

In addition to denial, other common defense mechanisms include **reaction formation** and **undoing** (Busch et al., 1995; A. Freud, 1936), both similarly utilized in the management of difficult-to-tolerate ambivalence and separation fears. Reaction formation involves the conversion of feelings into their opposite, such as anger into excessive caring. Rather than acknowledge anger at someone with whom they are having problems, individuals make extra efforts to help them, easing underlying fears that anger will damage or disrupt the relationship. In the defense of undoing, an individual makes amends for the conscious experience or outward expression of a conflicted wish or fantasy, usually an angry one. For example, patients may "take back" angry comments they have made, reassuring themselves and others that the aggression is not excessive or damaging. For example, a patient might say, "I feel my husband's been acting like a jerk, but I really do care about him."

Somatization is a common defense in a variety of disorders, as unacceptable feelings and fantasies are experienced as bodily events rather than as emotional ones. Physical symptoms can also symbolize an unconscious fantasy. The therapist works to identify the meanings and feelings that somatic symptoms are attempting to ward off or represent so that the patient and therapist can more effectively address them.

The treatment of Mr. A illustrates the unconscious use of defense mechanisms in his attempt to manage frightening angry feelings and fantasies.

CASE EXAMPLE: MR. A

Mr. A demonstrated the use of several defense mechanisms in conflicts about angry feelings and fantasies with his husband. He initially **denied** being angry at Joseph but, on further questioning, acknowledged some "frustration," being wary about using the word "anger." In addition, he suggested that his husband was only wanting to help him by trying to structure his day, so he was showing his concern; Mr. A was therefore not angry about his intrusiveness, a form of **reaction formation**. As he began to acknowledge his anger, he would often take it back, a form of **undoing**. For instance, he would say, "I guess I find it really irritating when Joe comes to bug me about what I should be doing to take better care of myself. Then again, I know he's just trying to help me." The use of these defenses provided opportunities for the therapist to point out to Mr. A that he was wary of his angry feelings and had various strategies for suppressing them. These observations helped him to gain greater access to these feelings and fantasies, enabling him to feel less threatened and manage them better.

Compromise Formation

A **compromise formation** (Freud, 1893–1895) is a fantasy, symptom, or behavior that symbolically expresses a compromise between an unacceptable wish and the defense against that wish. For example, panic attacks and other anxiety symptoms often represent a compromise between unacceptable or frightening aggressive fantasies, conflicted dependency wishes, and self-punishment for these fantasies. The aggressive wishes may emerge in a patient's efforts to coerce others to manage their anxiety and yet are minimized by that patient's presentation of being weak and in need of help. Unacceptable dependency wishes can also be expressed in physical symptoms that the patient experiences and communicates to others as being dangerous. The patient's terror can also function as self-punishment for conflicted wishes that trigger guilty feelings.

CASE EXAMPLE: MR. A

Mr. A's panic attacks expressed anger indirectly by his preoccupation with his symptoms, such as being fearful of having a heart attack, leaving his husband feeling more alone and emotionally isolated. The symptoms also expressed unacknowledged wishes to be taken care of at the same time that he was frustrated by his husband's intrusiveness. Finally, his frightening symptoms functioned as punishment for his angry feelings. Identification of these various functions helped to gain an understanding and better control over the multiple contributors to his panic attacks.

Unsymbolized States

Another set of feelings and fantasies are unsymbolized—that is, have not been identified in terms of verbal understanding. These internal states are often experienced as emerging from the body, or somatically. In addition to performing a defensive function, as described above, bodily reactions of anger and anxiety can be misidentified as a physical problem, sometimes believed to be catastrophic. The goal in treatment is to translate these phenomena into the language of feelings and fantasies, where they can be identified and worked with psychotherapeutically.

CASE EXAMPLE: MR. A

Mr. A experienced significant somatic symptoms that he believed were indicators of a serious medical situation, such as a heart attack. The therapist explained that, as his shortness of breath and chest pain were not evidence of an impending catastrophe, based on an exam by his internist that did not identify any medical problems, they had psychological meanings. Over the course of therapy, Mr. A learned that his focus on the body (somatic states) could function as a defense against his angry feelings and fantasies. In addition, bodily symptoms in part represented a compromise formation, a way of seeing himself as ill to reduce the threat from his aggression.

In addition to these functions around intrapsychic conflict, the therapist and Mr. A began to recognize that his somatic experiences also represented unidentified emotional states, specifically anxiety and anger. This understanding helped Mr. A to recognize how he often experienced his anger as anxiety, enabling him to better identify when he was irritated with Joseph or others.

Representations of Self and Others

Individuals have internalized (inner mental) **representations of themselves and of others,** derived primarily from significant early relationships (Bowlby, 1973; Jacobson, 1964). These internalized models exert ongoing significant influence and shape perceptions and expectations of self and others, often without awareness. The nature of these representations plays an important role in the development and emergence of symptoms and problems. Clinical and research evidence suggests that patients who have internalized representations of others predominantly involving criticism, rejection, attack, and/or intrusion are vulnerable to developing negative self-views and a variety of problems and disorders. For example, based on representations of others as frightening, temperamental, and judgmental (Arrindell et al., 1983; Parker, 1979; Silove, 1986), panic patients often anticipate that their relationships will be easily disrupted and that a range of feelings and experiences, particularly surrounding separation and anger, are unsafe. The following case demonstrates the powerful influence of internal representations on anxiety onset and persistence.

CASE EXAMPLE: MS. B

Ms. B, a 56-year-old White divorced woman who reported a long history of panic disorder, sought treatment for a recurrence of panic attacks. In the initial evaluation, the therapist identified that her panic was triggered by the idea of returning to work as an administrator in the financial industry after having been unemployed for many years. She described being frightened about interacting with male superiors on her return, worrying that she would be criticized about her intelligence or get fired. She believed her panic made sense given the circumstances and that it was caused by realistic concerns. Upon exploring her previous work experiences, she revealed that these had been primarily positive, with her bosses viewing her as competent. The therapist pointed out that, given her prior work success, her fears of male bosses appeared to be overstated, and it was important to understand what contributed to this exaggeration. The therapist recommended that she enter twice-weekly problem-focused psychodynamic psychotherapy in an effort to reassess her feelings and fantasies of danger that led to panic attacks.

Exploration of her past revealed that Ms. B had recurrent experiences with judgmental and temperamental men, including her father and husband. Her father had been intrusive and critical of her, particularly when he drank heavily, and the therapist suggested that this history contributed to her expectations that bosses would be rejecting and see her as inadequate. Indeed, her father verbally attacked her mother as incompetent and needy, and either ignored the patient or criticized her for being "stupid." A similar pattern arose in her relationship with her husband, who had episodes of insulting and rejecting her. He criticized her for complaining that he spent too much time at work, and after particularly intense fights, he would leave home, sometimes for extended periods. Ms. B feared confronting him about his behavior or his whereabouts, fearing he would abandon her permanently. Over the course of this relationship, the patient struggled with recurrent panic attacks, which improved when they divorced 10 years previously.

The therapist interpreted these experiences as having led her to develop internalized representations of men as critical and rejecting, causing her to anticipate being abused by them. Understanding these relationships and self and other representations and expectations helped the therapist and patient address her terror of men on returning to work, easing her panic symptoms.

Mentalization

Mentalization is the capacity to conceive of and interpret behaviors and motives in self and others in terms of mental states (Busch, 2008; Fonagy & Target, 1997). Therapists work to determine mentalization difficulties that contribute to specific problems. Mentalization is most likely to be disrupted in the context of intense attachment relationships, impairing the ability to communicate about needs and wishes. Many problems result from a misinterpretation of the behavior of others or anticipation of certain actions and attitudes. An improved comprehension of the motives and communication of others can aid in relief of these problems. For instance, patients who experience critical behavior from others can be helped by recognizing that others may be acting on the basis of their own emotions or stresses rather than a difficulty of the patient's.

CASE EXAMPLE: MR. A

In his ongoing efforts to address Mr. A's tensions with his husband, the therapist discussed with him what Joseph might be feeling in the way that he dealt with the patient. He began to recognize that Joseph was anxious about how Mr. A was doing and would respond to this with efforts to pressure the patient to have a more structured lifestyle. This realization further helped Mr. A to work with his frustration with his husband. He was able to have a productive discussion with Joseph, indicating that Joseph's approach made Mr. A more anxious rather than helped the situation, further easing the tensions between them and his panic symptoms.

CLINICAL MANIFESTATIONS

Symptoms

According to psychoanalytic theory, **symptoms** derive in part from the threatened emergence into consciousness of frightening or unacceptable unconscious feelings and fantasies (Freud, 1926). The conflicted unconscious content triggers anxiety, guilt, and the operation of defense mechanisms. Symptoms can represent compromise formations between the expression of a forbidden wish and the defense against that wish. Thus, symptoms are viewed as carrying important meanings and symbolize central conflicted fantasies and feelings. Several dynamic factors may contribute to specific symptoms or problems. For example, depressive symptoms of low motivation and self-criticism can represent conflicted aggression directed toward the self, a form of self-punishment, and a message to others that one is not an aggressive threat.

In identifying and designating problems, the therapist communicates that they have particular meanings and functions for patients, which are often maladaptive. Thus, defining problems and early exploration of context and feelings are methods for establishing symbolization. For example, the therapist clarifies that somatic symptoms have a psychological and emotional basis and therefore have a meaning for the patient. Bodily experiences can represent poorly symbolized emotions, a defense against painful feelings and fantasies, or a symbolized representation of an intrapsychic conflict, often involving dependency or aggression. In designating the somatic states as a symptom, the therapist suggests that understanding their meanings and functions will contribute to relief. The process of identifying symptoms, behaviors, and relationship difficulties as meaningful problems is a core part of this therapy.

CASE EXAMPLE: MS. C

Ms. C, a 45-year-old White married software engineer, described panic and anxiety symptoms that occurred primarily at work. The symptoms included chest pain, dizziness, and fears of falling down because she had "nothing to hold on to," and an experience of depersonalization, "not being sure who I am." She found her job dehumanizing and believed that the bosses disregarded the needs of their employees, viewing them as automatons. She was angry at the rigidity of the rules at work, such as the monitoring of time spent out of the office. She experienced her own boss as intrusive, critical, and demanding, creating significant anxiety. Her boss repeatedly questioned her about the status of projects, suggesting that Ms. C's pace was inadequate. She viewed her boss as rigid and incompetent and believed it was unfair that she should have to answer to him.

On the other hand, she worried that if she registered any of her complaints, she would be "being a bitch" and thought this could result in retaliation, including threats to her job.

In therapy, Ms. C described growing up in a critical and demanding family and agreed with the therapist that this likely related to her anxiety. She was the youngest child, and when she was a young adolescent, she was the only one still spending significant time with her mother, whose increasingly severe alcohol use led to her being regularly drunk during the day. During these periods, her mother was verbally abusive, calling Ms. C "fat" and "a burden." Ms. C worried that if she fought with her mother, it would trigger a more vicious assault. She was also fearful that her mother would get injured from being intoxicated and found herself spending more time at home to protect her.

Several underlying emotional factors were found to contribute to the onset of severe anxiety and panic attacks. These factors included intense fears of expressing her anger at her boss and potentially disrupting their relationship, fears that were found to mirror her early struggles with her mother. Ms. C's panic symptoms of feeling that there was "nothing to hold on to" and not being sure who she was were related to her mother's lack of support and recognition of her needs. These various intrapsychic dangers were displaced onto bodily concerns, including dizziness and chest pain. Thus, the therapist and patient identified the psychological meanings of her somatic symptoms. Recognition of how these various factors contributed to panic attacks, and that panic did not indicate current catastrophic dangers, aided in the reduction of her symptoms and associated problems, including her fears of assertiveness.

Resistance

Resistance refers to the patient's often unconscious efforts to thwart the therapeutic effects of the treatment to avoid the emergence of threatening or frightening feelings and fantasies, or to maintain an attachment to aspects of problems (e.g., having others take care of the patient) (Stone, 1973). This phenomenon may take several forms, including more overt behaviors, such as forgetting or coming late to appointments, expressly refusing to discuss a topic, or doing something self-destructive after making progress.

In psychoanalytic treatments, resistance can serve as a therapeutic marker, an indicator that the therapy is approaching threatening or conflicted unconscious fantasies or difficult feelings or topics. The therapist can demonstrate to the patient the nature of the resistance and suggest that the patient is avoiding something that appears to be important and threatening. An increase in resistance can also occur and be addressed when conflicted feelings and fantasies emerge with the therapist (see transference below). Although resistance is an important concept, the therapist should avoid using the term in therapy, such as saying to the patient "You're resisting . . . ," as it could be experienced as judgmental (see the therapist's interpretation below).

CASE EXAMPLE: MS. B

Ms. B became angry with the therapist after the third session of her treatment, when the therapist informed her of his upcoming vacation. It emerged that Ms. B believed that the 24 sessions of the protocol of which she was part needed to take place in 12 consecutive weeks, even though she had never been told this. She felt humiliated and stupid that she had made changes to her plans to accommodate something that was unnecessary. The therapist suggested that this transference response was consistent with Ms. B's proneness to feel humiliated and attack herself rather than direct her anger toward others. She unconsciously had imagined herself in a position of being poorly treated, as she anticipated with her future boss. Ms. B then demonstrated resistance, as she shifted to minimizing her reaction, saying that this incident was "no biggie" and that she actually did not feel strongly about the misunderstanding. The therapist suggested to the patient that she may be taking back the painful emotions she had described because they were threatening to her. Although she initially brushed aside the therapist's interpretation, in subsequent sessions Ms. B acknowledged her hurt and frustration. She described a pattern of experiencing an anxious pressure to accommodate others, followed by anger, humiliation, and self-criticism about being overly yielding.

Regression

The term **regression** describes a shift in cognition, emotions, and often behavior to an earlier developmental level (Arlow, 1963; Freud, 1917). Regression can affect thoughts, feelings, self and other representations, and fantasies. Regression can occur in response to intrapsychic conflicts, especially in response to threats arising from autonomy, assertiveness, separation, and loss. For example, panic, anxiety, and depressive disorders may involve a regressed state of needy, helpless behavior to minimize threats from aggressive feelings and fantasies. This behavior, along with a focus on bodily symptoms, can also express dependency wishes that are otherwise unacceptable or generate fears of rejection.

CASE EXAMPLE: MS. D

Ms. D was a 28-year-old Asian woman suffering from depressive symptoms, living at home with her mother. She described her mother as cooking and cleaning for her, as she barely made efforts to care for herself, spending much of her time on social media or watching movies. Ms. D had recently graduated from business school but was deeply dispirited by her performance there. Although her grades were good, she was angry and depressed that she did not receive honors. She also did not obtain a highly prized internship that she had sought.

Following these disappointments, which she referred to as failures, she developed a surge of depressive symptoms, including down mood, intense self-criticism, and decreased motivation. She was not applying for jobs or doing any networking. Following a consultation, her therapist began a trial of escitalopram, an antidepressant. He also recommended PrFPP, as it was important to understand why Ms. D viewed these events as failures rather than disappointments.

In exploring her developmental history, it emerged that her father had been a driven perfectionistic businessman who had high academic and professional expectations of the patient and her brother. When she was 16 years old, he left her mother for a younger woman. The woman, who subsequently became her stepmother, deeply discouraged contact with his children, which became minimal. The patient had a fantasy that if she became highly successful, he would invest more interest in her, and that now she had failed to achieve that goal. Her regression and depression indicated the pain around his loss of interest and that now the only way to gain love and attention was to be helpless and taken care of by her mother. It also emerged that Ms. D was deeply conflicted about anger at her mother for having lost her father's affection and that her helpless regressed state also represented a defense against this anger. Exploring these contributory factors aided the patient in recognizing the self-destructiveness of her regression, the excessiveness of her self-criticism, and the need to address fears of moving forward in her life.

Transference

Emotions and perceptions that develop from prior significant relationships, particularly in early life, emerge in all relationships, including with the therapist, a phenomenon referred to as **transference** (Freud, 1905). The therapist helps patients to articulate feelings, fantasies, and conflicts that emerge in the therapeutic relationship. The transference provides a directness and immediacy in recognizing and understanding conflicted emotions and fantasies as they come to life with the therapist. The therapist's nonjudgmental stance in response to patients' feelings and expressions is crucial in providing a sense of safety for unconscious mental states to emerge, as patients typically anticipate a critical, intrusive, or unempathic response. This stance also helps to ease patients' guilt and shame about what they are communicating to the therapist and increase their sense of trust.

Interpreting the transference also helps identify patients' self and other representations, including the characteristic ways in which they misperceive others and how these perceptions generalize to other relationships (see Cooper, 1987; Westen & Gabbard, 2002). Patients' increased awareness of feelings, conflicts, defenses, and actions obtained via the transference provides valuable information in building a psychodynamic formulation and addressing problems. Emotions and conflicts regarding the therapist can help to identify specific triggers of problems, such as a patient's feeling injured or becoming angry. For instance, angry feelings typically develop toward the therapist in the setting of vacations or termination, along with fears about losing or disrupting the relationship with the therapist. These separations provide important opportunities for patients to better articulate, understand, and manage their conflicts about anger and autonomy in the setting of the transference.

Sometimes patients enact their issues behaviorally rather than verbally in what is referred to as **acting in**. For instance, patients may come late to appointments or delay payment of bills. They may miss or "forget" a session after discussing a difficult topic or avoid raising an issue that they are frustrated about. Exploring these behaviors provides additional opportunities to examine problems in the context of the transference relationship, with more direct access to triggering cues, feelings, and conflicts.

CASE EXAMPLE: MR. E

Mr. E, a 46-year-old White business executive, struggled with surges of anger alternating with anxiety and depression, particularly after his wife asked for a divorce. He reported extensive bullying by his father, leading him to develop chronic fears of asserting himself alternating with episodes of rage at what he believed was others taking advantage of him. His transference to the therapist mirrored that of his experience of his father, viewing the therapist as rigid and controlling, with an intention to dominate or humiliate the patient. For instance, he expressed fury at the therapist for ending sessions in a timely manner but then feared the therapist would retaliate against him for expressing these feelings. The therapist identified how Mr. E was perceiving him to be like his father, even though the therapist did not intend to control or humiliate him. This interpretation helped the patient understand how he expected the therapist, and others in his life, to attack and reject him like his father, increasing his anxiety and anger.

Countertransference

Therapists develop reactions to patients based on their own experiences, conflicts, and self and other representations, referred to as **countertransference** (Gabbard, 1995). Therapists' alertness to their countertransference can help them avoid problematic reactions to patients that can interfere with treatment, such as being drawn into patients' sense of urgency or struggling with guilt about going on vacation. However, countertransference can also be a useful clinical tool, aiding therapists in identifying patients' feelings, fantasies, and transference. Therapists can become more aware of particular countertransferences to which they are prone through their own therapy and by self-monitoring (Gabbard, 1995; Sandler, 1976). For example, a therapist who had traumatic experiences of abandonment and felt hurt and angry when patients canceled sessions needed to learn how to appropriately manage those feelings. Countertransference can also provide information about what kinds of interpersonal problems patients may be prone to by provoking or inducing certain types of reactions in others.

Psychoanalysts in the school of relational analysis (see below) emphasize the interpersonal field as a core component of the ongoing analytic process. The relationship is explored in terms of the transference/countertransference aspects of the treatment. The analyst communicates about these factors with patients in a way that helps them understand their internal conflicts and relationship problems.

CASE EXAMPLE: MS. B

When Ms. B minimized her reaction to the therapist's vacation schedule, the therapist became aware of urges to argue with her to get her to recognize the similarity of the transference situation to the conflicts she experienced. Fearing criticism and rejection, Ms. B's expectations of herself and others led her to anticipate others' demands and respond to them. This pattern, which occurred with job seeking and men in positions of authority, led her to recurrently feel anxious, angry, and humiliated. However, efforts to get her to accept this dynamic in the transference were met with increased resistance from Ms. B, averring that the therapist was making a "big deal of nothing." The therapist recognized that his urge to argue with this patient was unusual for him and that he risked behaving in a way that would create precisely the situation the patient feared—being pressured by a man (see enactments below). This recognition also helped him become aware of the intensity of Ms. B's avoidance of these feelings. The therapist stopped pursuing this topic, allowing Ms. B to more safely explore the threats of humiliation she anticipated with others before returning to their relationship.

Enactments

Sometimes patients' dynamics and problems interact with the therapist's countertransference to create what is referred to as enactments (Cassorla, 2013). For instance, the therapist may avoid exploring painful traumatic experiences due to the distress it causes the therapist, and the patient may sense the therapist's reaction and avoid those topics. It is important for therapists to be alert to behaviors or feelings that are unusual for them, so they can identify potential enactments (e.g., getting into a power struggle with the patient). Therapists should explore what is happening with the patient that is triggering this reaction to help them out of the enactment and use this information to better address dynamics and problems.

CASE EXAMPLE: MR. E

An example of an enactment occurred when Mr. E began to constantly challenge the frame of the treatment. He would often arrive at the session a few minutes late and then express rage that the therapist would end the session on time. He snarled that this was unfair and demonstrated the therapist's rigidity and "mercenary" tendencies.

Frequently, he would declare the session a waste of time. The therapist worked to identify the patient's wish for control and his misreading of the boundaries of treatment as the therapist's effort to humiliate him. At the same time, the therapist felt bullied by Mr. E's pressure to shift the boundaries. The therapist noticed that he was increasingly frustrated with the patient and on occasion would withhold comments that he thought might help Mr. E settle down. Recognizing the enactment and considering how best to handle it, the therapist suggested that the patient was reenacting the struggle with his father rather than learning from it. Why not make more of an effort to come on time? The patient was annoyed about this suggestion but shifted his behavior, improving the immediate conflict with the therapist and the therapeutic process.

PSYCHOANALYTIC MODELS OF THE MIND

This book uses four predominant psychoanalytic models of the mind as theories and approaches to treatment. They include symbolization models, object relations theory, conflict/defense theory, and relational/interpersonal conceptions.

Symbolization Models

Symbolization models involve various ways that presymbolic or dissociated states (see box below) become translated into symbolized mental content, contributing building blocks to other aspects of intrapsychic and interpersonal functioning and behavior. Presymbolic states include drives, affects (differentiated from symbolized emotions), somatic experiences, and dissociated states (Bucci, 1997; Isaacs, 1948). Techniques used to aid the symbolization process include verbalizing, defining, and linking emotions, somatic states, and impulses to self and other representations and environmental events (Busch, 2017).

SYMBOLIZATION OF UNMENTALIZED STATES

Contents: Affects/somatic experiences; drives/urges; dissociated states

Pathology: Unsymbolized and dissociated states emerge in affective surges, impulses, and somatic symptoms

Goals: Symbolization/mentalization: convert unmentalized states to usable, thinkable experience and information

Techniques: Define and link affective and somatic states, urges, and self and other representations; interpret defensive functions that maintain unsymbolized states

Object Relations Theory

This category consists of self and other representations along with accompanying emotions. Self/other units impact perception and prediction, potentially creating a distortion of self and other expectations (i.e., self-criticism, rejection, or negative judgments by others). Techniques include identification of self and other representations (see box below) and how they influence current experiences and symptoms, and challenging adverse perceptions of self and others.

> ### SELF/OTHER REPRESENTATIONS
>
> **Contents:** Symbolized self and other representations with accompanying emotions
>
> **Pathology:** Inaccurate self and other perceptions and expectations, including intensely negative self-views or expectations of damaging or being damaged or abandoned by others
>
> **Goals:** Recognition of self and other representations that operate out of awareness; less negative self and other representations; and increased flexibility of representations, with greater accuracy to current reality
>
> **Techniques:** Clarify self and other representations and accompanying emotions; identify conflicted self and other representations and emotions; correct negative self and other representations via actual experiences with others, including in the transference

Conflict/Defense Theory

This model describes unconscious or emerging conscious wishes and fantasies that feel intolerable or unacceptable, causing guilt and anxiety. Defense mechanisms are triggered to prevent these wishes from becoming conscious and manage the guilt and anxiety these wishes create (A. Freud, 1936). Defenses may also operate by disrupting symbolization to protect the individual from identifying painful feelings and fantasies. For example, somatization can function as a regressive defense to prevent the awareness of certain feelings or fantasies, such as those involving anger or longings for others. Conflicts and defenses (see box below) often combine in the form of compromise formations. The therapist works with the patient to identify defense mechanisms, compromise formations, and underlying conflicted wishes as they emerge, including in the transference.

> ### INTRAPSYCHIC CONFLICTS AND DEFENSES
>
> **Contents:** Wishes/fantasies that are felt to be intolerable, unacceptable, or dangerous; defense mechanisms that are triggered to prevent these fantasies and wishes, or

unmentalized contents, from becoming conscious, attempting to manage guilt and anxiety; development of compromise formations

Pathology: Conflicts about unconscious/conscious wishes that create guilt, shame, and anxiety; defense mechanisms that are triggered and can create rigidity and be experienced as symptoms; symptoms that represent compromise formations between wishes and defenses

Goals: Increase awareness/tolerance of emotions/wishes/intrapsychic conflicts; recognize that fantasies are not as dangerous as anticipated if not enacted or expressed appropriately; interpret defenses and symptoms to help identify intrapsychic conflicts; reduce guilt, anxiety, and other symptoms

Techniques: Interpret defenses to help gain access to conflicted wishes and fantasies; identify conflicted wishes and fantasies, which enables reassessment of the sense of danger and intolerability associated with them; clarify defenses and conflicted wishes as they emerge in the transference; relieve symptoms as the intrapsychic conflicts and defenses that contribute to them become conscious and are reassessed

Relational/Interpersonal Conceptions

This model addresses actual interaction (verbal, nonverbal) or communication about the interaction between self and others (Mitchell, 1988). Self/other interactions regulate affects and shape self and other representations. The therapist works to identify and communicate the nature of these interpersonal experiences with the patient, including enactments and disruptions in the therapeutic relationship (see box below). This information is also used to identify and address dissociated self-states. The therapist examines transference and countertransference to aid in elaborating the interpersonal field created by both parties, informed by each of their histories (Stern, 2015). Techniques include metacommunication about interactions, identifying countertransference/transference states, denoting and addressing enactments, and addressing disruptions in the therapeutic relationship.

RELATIONAL/INTERPERSONAL FACTORS

Contents: Interactions between self and others; addressing of these experiences; units of the interpersonal field, including self in interaction with the other; elements include verbal and behavioral interactions, reactions triggered in others, and nonverbal communication

Pathology: Co-constructed relationship difficulties, enactments, dissociated self and other representations, and relationship disruptions

Goals: Identify dissociated self and other representations; identify, translate, and reduce enactments; reduce co-constructed problematic interactions, disruptions

> **Techniques:** Identify countertransference/transference states; metacommunication; denote and address enactments; address disruptions in the therapeutic relationship

CONCLUSION

With these definitions in mind, we now proceed to explore how these concepts guide the psychodynamic formulation and intervention in a problem-focused psychodynamic psychotherapy.

> **QUESTIONS AND IDEAS TO THINK ABOUT**
>
> 1. Considering a patient in your current practice, think about what intrapsychic conflicts and defenses, negative self and other representations, and mentalization disruptions this patient struggles with and how they relate to the problems you are treating.
> 2. Considering a patient in your practice, think about what symptoms, resistance, and transference issues this patient contends with. What countertransference reactions might you have toward this patient?

CHAPTER 2

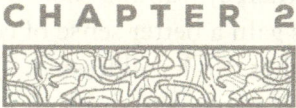

Identifying Problems

As discussed briefly in Chapter 1, the identification of specific problems is a key therapeutic task of problem-focused psychodynamic psychotherapy (PrFPP; Busch, 2022). A set of core problems are identified early in the treatment, but others may emerge subsequently. Patients will report some problems as active sources of distress, whereas others are out of awareness or operate reflexively, taking more time to be recognized. Other problems come to light after barriers that obscure or hide them, such as shame, denial, or other defenses, are addressed. This chapter describes how the therapist goes about identifying the specific nature of the patient's problems, including the thoughts, feelings, and circumstances that accompany them, as well as how the therapist can address barriers that interfere with that identification. The chapter concludes with information on how to develop a problem list that can be used to maintain focus as the treatment proceeds with identifying relevant psychodynamic contributors and interventions.

DEVELOPING SELF-REFLECTIVE SKILLS

The initial efforts in PrFPP not only designate problems that become the focus of treatment, but also engage patients in the process of stepping back and exploring their difficulties, developing self-observational skills (described in greater depth in Chapter 3). As therapists ask guiding questions to identify the details, triggers, and contexts of problems, this exploratory process helps patients improve their capacity to attend to their own thoughts, feelings, and motivations. Patients can therefore begin to recognize that certain emotions, thoughts, behaviors, and situations contribute to their problems. This approach also helps patients see problems as distinct rather than as an inherent part of themselves or caused by others, thereby framing them as something that potentially can be relieved. In addition, patients gain a better sense of control by recognizing that problems have specific contributors that can be addressed. The guiding questions described throughout this chapter encourage patients to think about situations, thoughts, and emotions that trigger or exacerbate problems. As is demonstrated in these cases, individual problems have unique features, triggers, and histories for patients that provide information that will be used to address and relieve them.

In the initial session or two, you want to give the patient a clear view of how you envision the therapy progressing. The educational handout provided at the end of this chapter (Handout 2.1, p. 42) can be given to patients to provide an overview of the treatment. (For your convenience, a downloadable version of this handout is available online at *www.guilford.com/busch-forms*.)

TYPES OF PROBLEMS

For the purposes of the PrFPP approach, problems are divided into symptoms, behavioral difficulties, personality issues, and relationship struggles. Each of these categories is used in elaborating a problem list but should not be seen as starkly discrete, as problem areas can overlap. Unassertiveness, for example, can be experienced in the form of symptoms, behavioral problems, or relationship difficulties. It is not essential, however, to clearly categorize a problem. The therapist and patient will define the language and components of problems in terms that are comprehensible for the patient. In some circumstances, a shorthand term can be useful in alluding to specific problems, such as "your depression," "your intense self-criticism," "your conflicts with your spouse," or "your difficulty controlling your temper."

The initial question set that follows here elicits information about the primary problem or problems patients are struggling with. As we move through the chapter, other guiding question sets are presented that are used to screen for the various categories of problems described above. Later, still other guiding questions are presented that seek to address problems that patients may hesitate to discuss because of guilt or shame, as well as other issues that they do not recognize as problems. You can use the questions as a guide for your clinical interview, or you can give patients the worksheet, saying, "Before our next session, I'd like you to try completing this worksheet. It asks you to describe the problems you have, including the history of them and the triggers that contribute to them."

Identifying the Patient's Presenting Problems

The guiding questions asked by the therapist in the case that follows here (of Mr. F) represent an initial step in obtaining information about the patient's problems, including associated thoughts and feelings, history, severity, and triggers.

Identifying Problems 25

For convenience, these questions are organized into Worksheet 2.1: Initial Identification of Problems (pp. 43–44; see *www.guilford.com/busch-forms*). As with all the guiding questions presented in the book, those that follow are offered as a guide for your work in session with the patient. But they are not intended as a rigid script to follow, as you may need to modify or adjust them based on the responses of the patient.

CASE EXAMPLE: MR. F'S COMPULSIVE BEHAVIOR

Mr. F, a 37-year-old White personal accountant, presented with feelings of intolerable pressure and anxiety at his job, which required him to work long hours and disrupted his relationship with his family. It emerged that he could readily reduce his workload by turning down new cases, but he felt compelled to accept each new referral. The work stress was so severe that he would be distracted during phone or zoom meetings with clients by unrelated paperwork that needed to be completed and would sometimes lose track of what they were saying. At first, he denied that this distraction and divided attention were an issue, but he soon acknowledged that he was worried about making an error or being "caught" by a client because he was focusing on something else. A key question that emerged in his treatment was why the patient put himself under this enormous pressure.

THERAPIST: How would you describe the main concerns or problems that brought you in for therapy?

MR. F: I guess I'd call my problem **overwork**. I get very stressed and **anxious** about completing what I need to do each day. I'm terrified my clients are going to get angry that I haven't finished their taxes. And then I run into **problems with my wife**. She's furious that I don't get home sooner and help more with the kids. I mean I'm the one earning the money, and I feel she should have a little more respect for what I'm doing.

THERAPIST: How severe are these problems? How much are they disrupting your life?

MR. F: They're definitely causing a lot of disruptions. I'm anxious much of the time, and the fights with my wife are a big source of tension.

THERAPIST: Do you believe there are triggers of these problems? If so, what might they be?

MR. F: I'm not sure. I've always felt pressure to work hard. Going way back to when I was in school. Somehow, I've always felt like I'm not accomplishing enough. Maybe because my father put a lot of pressure on me? I don't know. And my overwork then seems to set off all the other problems.

THERAPIST: What was going on in your life when you started having these problems? What were the various stresses in your life at that time? Are they still present?

MR. F: It worsened about 10 years ago, when I started my practice, and we also had our first child. I guess I felt more pressure when we had our third child a year ago. My wife feels I should contribute more to child care, even though I do more than a lot of fathers I know. Also, I have some **financial pressure**. We bought a new house when we had our third child and maybe we bit off a bit more than we can chew. I certainly think about that when I consider turning down a client.

THERAPIST: Do you notice anything that happens or any thoughts or feelings you have just before your symptoms or problems get worse or return?

MR. F: I know when I think to myself you shouldn't take on another case, I start to feel lazy, and I feel anxious about not being busy enough or making enough money. Then if I do take the case, I feel anxious about that! Like, how am I going to get all this work done?

THERAPIST: Are there any other problems you've been having?

MR. F: I have the worries about money and the conflicts with my wife. I've also had a bit of a flirtation at the office. I feel guilty about it sometimes, but other times I feel I deserve more positive attention because I get so much trouble from my wife. It's pretty exciting. I mean nothing's happened yet, but we've talked about how we feel about each other. Oh, and my wife thinks I **drink too much**, but I don't think that's an issue for me.

Symptoms

When identifying symptoms, the therapist explores their severity and pervasiveness, circumstances in which they emerge, feelings and thoughts that accompany them, their history, and potential triggers. The following sections present guiding questions for evaluation of anxiety, depression, and somatic symptoms. (For your convenience, these sets of questions are also available in a variety of worksheets that you can download and use at *www.guilford.com/busch-forms*.) These guiding questions are not intended to be full evaluations of these various symptoms and disorders and are not meant to replace more complete clinical evaluation and systematic assessment tools. Their intent is to demonstrate how to define problems in PrFPP and begin to become aware of their triggers and contributors to them.

Initial Evaluation of Anxiety

The discussion that follows in the case of Ms. G uses the guiding questions in Worksheet 2.2: Initial Evaluation of Anxiety (pp. 45–46).

CASE EXAMPLE: MS. G'S ANXIETY

Ms. G was a 24-year-old White single woman paralegal presenting for treatment of anxiety. She initially described her primary problem as social anxiety. However, it emerged that she experienced anxiety in a much broader range of situations.

Identifying Problems

THERAPIST: Have you been experiencing anxiety?

MS. G: Yes, I would definitely say anxiety is my main problem.

THERAPIST: How severe has it been?

MS. G: Pretty severe. Sometimes I even avoid going to a social event because of the worry it's causing me.

THERAPIST: How frequently do you experience anxiety? Do you feel it much of the time or only occasionally?

MS. G: I guess all told I'm anxious pretty frequently. In addition to social anxiety, I worry about my health and about being alone at night. It starts to add up.

THERAPIST: What kinds of circumstances trigger your anxiety?

MS. G: I'm anxious to some degree in all social situations but much worse at a group activity. I get worried even when I think about going to a party. I try to figure out who will be there and how they might react to me. I might be preoccupied with it for a whole day before I go. But it can happen in almost any situation where I'm in front of a group. Let's say I have to give a speech. I get embarrassed and feel I'll be judged. I worry about saying something stupid and that others will criticize me.

THERAPIST: What kinds of thoughts accompany your anxiety? Can you describe them?

MS. G: I start thinking about whether this person is judging me. Did I just say something dumb? Or perhaps I said something insulting. I get so anxious that sometimes it's hard for me to talk at all. Then I feel worse. Like now they'll really judge me for not having anything to say. I can also become very anxious about having a disease. Sort of like a hypochondriac. I get a cough and worry it's cancer. And I get scared when I'm in my house alone at night that someone's going to break in and attack me, even though I live in a really safe neighborhood and I've never heard of this happening to anyone.

THERAPIST: When did your anxiety start? What was going on in your life at that time?

MS. G: I've felt anxious for a long time, at least since adolescence. Maybe that's when I was getting more social. Also, that's when my parents started arguing more.

THERAPIST: Do you have panic attacks (episodes of severe anxiety accompanied by symptoms such as chest pain, shortness of breath, palpitations, catastrophic feelings of doom)? Do you notice any particular circumstances or thoughts and feelings that trigger your panic episodes?

MS. G: Yes. Sometimes I get panicky when I'm in a really scary social situation. My heart starts beating really rapidly, and I feel a bit shaky. One time, after I had a fight with my boyfriend, I had chest pain and thought I might be having a heart attack. But I was able to calm myself down by telling myself it was just anxiety.

Subsequently, the therapist explored the arguing between Ms. G's parents and the fight with her boyfriend as triggers of her fears. In addition, the therapist addressed her expectations of negative judgments by others in social situations.

Initial Evaluation of Depression

The discussion that follows in the case of Mr. H uses the guiding questions in Worksheet 2.3: Initial Evaluation of Depression (pp. 47–48).

CASE EXAMPLE: MR. H'S DEPRESSION

Mr. H was a 28-year-old gay White male graduate student who struggled with depressive symptoms for 6 months, after a breakup with his boyfriend.

THERAPIST: Have you felt down or depressed?

MR. H: I've felt down for about 6 months.

THERAPIST: How intense has your depression been?

MR. H: It's been pretty bad at times. Sometimes I just can't get any work done. I just lie in bed for hours. But I've never been suicidal or anything like that.

THERAPIST: Can you describe your symptoms?

MR. H: In addition to feeling down, my energy has been kind of low and I have trouble concentrating. I feel like my life is messed up and feel lonely.

THERAPIST: Have you noticed any triggers of your symptoms?

MR. H: One of them is pretty obvious. I broke up with my boyfriend about 6 months ago. That's when it started. And I guess my symptoms get worse when I'm alone. When I get together with friends, that can help.

THERAPIST: What kinds of thoughts and feelings do you have when you're down?

MR. H: I feel lonely. And I feel like a bad person. Like there's something wrong with me. Maybe I do something to drive people away.

THERAPIST: Do you get self-critical?

MR. H: I get really mad at myself for not getting things done. I feel I should be able to overcome my depression. And I think there's something wrong with me, like I have a mental illness. For example, I'm not really sure why I broke up with my boyfriend, who was actually a pretty good partner.

THERAPIST: Are there any other issues you believe are contributing to your depression?

MR. H: My family is in another country, so I feel kind of cut off from them. And we don't get along that well. They didn't handle my coming out too well. I don't get much support from them. Also, I'm not 100% sure what to do after graduate school. It's hard finding a job here. I need to consider going back to the country I'm from, but I'm not very excited about that prospect.

The therapist followed up by saying, "It sounds like there are several stresses that contributed to your depression that are important to explore. We also need to address your intense self-criticism, even about being depressed!"

Initial Evaluation of Somatic Symptoms

It is common for patients with psychological problems to experience bodily symptoms and have varying degrees of concern about them. *The discussion that follows in the case of Ms. I uses the guiding questions in Worksheet 2.4: Initial Evaluation of Somatic Symptoms (pp. 49–50) to elaborate the content of her somatic symptoms along with associated triggers, thoughts, and emotions.*

CASE EXAMPLE: MS. I'S SOMATIC SYMPTOMS

Ms. I was a 36-year-old Black administrative assistant presenting with worries about her health and her body that were preoccupying her and causing her significant distress.

THERAPIST: Do you have any concerns or worries about your body? If so, can you describe them?

MS. I: Yes, I definitely have that. For example, recently I've had bad headaches and I'm worried it might be a brain tumor.

THERAPIST: How long have you had these worries?

MS. I: For several weeks. But I've had worries about my health in the past.

THERAPIST: What was going on in your life when these worries started? Any particular stresses?

MS. I: Nothing that had anything to do with my headache. But I did have a terrible fight with my friend around the time it started. I found out she went out with another friend of ours that she's not even close to and she didn't even invite me!

THERAPIST: Have these stresses caused you significant distress?

MS. I: Yes, I'm thinking about it a lot! I'm so furious with her, and I can't believe she did that. I feel I'm on the bottom of everyone's list in terms of priority. But I'm afraid to talk to her because I'm so mad I'm worried what I might say to her. And then at the same time, I've been worrying about this headache.

THERAPIST: Have you had fears like this before? Were any stresses associated with those fears?

MS. I: I have. I mean every now and then I developed a fear that something was wrong with my health. I don't recall if I was stressed at the time. I mean I've had a lot of problems socially. I grew up in a small town, and I was very popular, but I've had a lot of problems with friends here. Nobody really sticks together, and a lot of times I get left out. And sometimes I feel I'm excluded because I'm Black. But I wouldn't do that to anyone else. I always try to include everyone.

THERAPIST: Have you been to the doctor about this problem or other concerns about your health? What have the doctors said?

MS. I: I haven't gone to them about this problem. But I've been to them before about my health worries. So far, they never found anything. One or two have said it was psychological. That's why I'm here seeing you!

The therapist commented that it felt important to talk about her feelings of being excluded by others, as those experiences appeared to be contributing to her anxiety.

Behavioral Problems

Although behavioral problems can come in many forms, two primary categories are areas of inhibition and areas of poor impulse control. Both benefit from identifying the behavioral problems and associated feelings, thoughts, and circumstances. In general, efforts to change behavior have been considered disruptive of psychodynamic psychotherapy, whereas in PrFPP, behavior is a target of treatment.

Initial Evaluation of Behavior Problems

For many patients, inhibitions arise and become problematic when they interfere with their life activities, whether occupational or social. In addition, inhibitions create difficulties when they prevent addressing issues in relationships. For example, Mr. A was inhibited about talking to his husband about their problems due to fears of creating tensions between them. Impulse control problems, on the other hand (see Ms. J), occur when individuals have difficulty managing behaviors that create difficulties for them, such as their temper, sexual impulses, drug use, eating, or shopping. Clinical examples of inhibitions and impulse control problems are presented throughout this book.

Refer to the guiding questions in Worksheet 2.5: Initial Evaluation of Inhibited Behaviors (pp. 51–52) and Worksheet 2.6: Initial Evaluation of Behaviors That Are Difficult to Control (pp. 53–54). The discussion that follows in the case of Ms. J uses the guiding questions in Worksheet 2.6.

CASE EXAMPLE: MS. J'S ANGRY SHOPPING

Ms. J, a 40-year-old saleswoman and mother of two, complained of significant anger at her husband. He had lost his job, and she felt he was making inadequate efforts to find a new one. She considered him a "downer," moping around the house while refusing to get help. In the initial evaluation, problems emerged with impulse control involving her shopping behavior.

THERAPIST: Do you have trouble controlling certain behaviors or impulses? Sexual wishes? Temper? Alcohol or drugs? Shopping?

MS. J: I do have problems with shopping. I mean I really love to shop. But my husband gets very angry with me and tells me I spend too much. Especially when the credit card bill comes in. But then I get furious with him for trying to stop me.

THERAPIST: Do you notice any triggers for this behavior?

MS. J: I tend to buy things when I'm mad. For example, when I'm mad at my husband. I'm so upset with how negative he is. I want to get some enjoyment. Or when I'm frustrated with work. I'm not treated very well by the guys there, and I don't think anybody credits me for what I do. I'll leave work at the end of the day and head straight to the store.

THERAPIST: When did these problems start? Were there any particular stresses in your life at that time?

MS. J: I've always had some trouble with shopping. But it got much worse 5 years ago, when my husband lost his job. And, you know, he's not really making any efforts to find a new one. I get so annoyed about it. And he wants to tell me what to do about the money?

THERAPIST: Do you feel guilty about these behaviors?

MS. J: Sometimes I do and sometimes I don't. I have the right to buy things because I make most of the money in the house. But then when he brings me the credit card bills and shows me what I've spent I have a wave of guilt.

THERAPIST: What are the consequences of these behaviors?

MS. J: As I've mentioned before, I get huge credit card bills, and my husband gets very upset. Sometimes I return things but then I just do it again.

THERAPIST: Have you tried to get control over these behaviors?

MS. J: Oh, definitely. After he shows me the credit cards, I promise him and myself that I'm going to cut back or stop buying expensive things. But then something frustrating happens, and sure enough I'm online or go into a store. I don't even think about the promise I made.

Personality Problems

Personality difficulties are a source of persistent problems for many individuals. Personality issues are typically not recognized by patients, as the attitudes and behaviors stemming from them are experienced as part of who they are. Patients may make such comments as "Others are always taking advantage of me," "Other people don't follow rules like I do," "I can't manage my life without others' support," or "I just don't get recognized for my skills." Additionally, patients can feel injured or threatened by designating a problem as part of their personality. Therefore, with personality issues, the therapist should work to identify the specific characteristics as part of the problem list in ways that are acceptable and comprehensible for patients. For example, problems with assertiveness, difficulties controlling impulses, and being avoidant of others are ways of describing personality factors that help patients acknowledge them. It can be difficult to directly obtain information about personality issues, as patients are unable to recognize them directly. However, the therapist should be alert to the emergence of these factors in the context of people describing their problems.

Personality issues span a range of problems and functional difficulties for patients. Personality disorders can be grouped into clusters that share common features (American Psychiatric Association, 2022). Cluster C disorders are characterized by anxious and fearful thoughts, feelings, and behavior. Avoidant personality disorder, for example, is characterized by social anxiety, fears of rejection, and feelings of inadequacy that lead to avoidance of a variety of situations, including social interactions.

Initial Evaluation of Avoidant Personality

What follows here is a continuation of the case of Ms. G. The guiding questions the therapist uses in this discussion are also available in the online Worksheet 2.7: Initial Evaluation of Avoidant Tendencies (p. 55).

CASE EXAMPLE: MS. G'S AVOIDANT PERSONALITY

Avoidant personality problems emerged in the context of exploring Ms. G's difficulties. It is common for avoidant tendencies to accompany anxiety disorders.

THERAPIST: Does your anxiety lead you to avoid certain situations?

MS. G: I have a lot of trouble asserting myself with people. I'm kind of a people pleaser. I'm very frightened of confrontation, so I avoid that entirely.

THERAPIST: How long have you had these avoidance problems?

MS. G: This goes way back to childhood. I've always been on the wary side and hesitant to confront people about problems. Otherwise, I'm worried they'll get angry at me.

THERAPIST: Are you aware of triggers of this avoidance or of situations that make it worse?

MS. G: It definitely gets worse with authority figures and people who are demanding. That's where it really gets scary. They're a bit like my father. He was a real "my way or the highway" kind of guy. But really, any social or work situation can be scary.

THERAPIST: What kinds of thoughts precede or accompany your fears and avoidance?

MS. G: I'm worried that other people aren't going to like me and that they're going to reject me if I raise any concerns. Even if I get frustrated about something, I'm frightened that if I bring it up, the other person will get really mad. For instance, my friend picks where we'll go for dinner, and if I want to go to a different place, I won't say anything. I worry she'll get furious, and we'll just end up doing what she wants anyway.

Evaluation of Narcissistic Personality Problems

Another cluster of personality disorders, Cluster B, involves dramatic or emotional behavior that can appear unpredictable. Within that cluster, narcissistic personality issues represent a particularly sensitive area for patients, as they likely do not recognize these traits as problematic and tend to view pointing out these characteristics as attacks and can be dismissive or angry in response. Although criteria for these disorders often emphasize feelings of superiority or entitlement, such individuals may be more willing to consider that they have a sensitivity to rejection or feel underrecognized by others, triggering anger, anxiety, and depression. If patients acknowledge these concerns, other narcissistic issues may be identified as reactions to these vulnerabilities. Thus, the therapist can suggest that a patient's sense of certainty or pressure to be "special" can represent an attempt to compensate for negative self-perceptions and fears of being undermined by others.

The following case of Mr. K uses the guiding questions based on the initial Worksheet 2.1 (pp. 43–44) to identify narcissistic issues.

CASE EXAMPLE: MR. K AND PATHOLOGICAL NARCISSISM

Mr. K was a 52-year-old Asian highly successful lawyer who presented with depressive symptoms after feeling frustrated and disappointed with his new job. He had presumed he would be a star employee there and instead struggled and felt unrecognized.

THERAPIST: How would you describe the main concerns or problems that brought you in for therapy?

MR. K: I left my law firm job and moved to a tech start-up that focused on legal services.

But from the start there, I wasn't recognized for my skill set or given a proper role in the company. I tried to return to my old firm, but they weren't interested anymore. I was shocked! I was a major rainmaker there!

THERAPIST: How severe are these problems? How much are they disrupting your life?

MR. K: I've had a very difficult time. I feel down and angry most of the time since I've been treated so badly.

THERAPIST: Do you believe there are triggers of these problems? If so, what might they be?

MR. K: Yes, whenever I have to deal with the idiots at my current firm. They put me in a new work group, and they don't really know what they're doing. And the firm isn't doing well because they didn't listen to me. When I think about looking for another job, I'm worried no one will be interested in me because now I'll be seen as a loser.

THERAPIST: What was going on in your life when you started having these problems? What were the various stresses in your life at that time? Are they still present?

MR. K: I've been frustrated since I've been at this new firm. It's been a year now. I'm working with a bunch of idiots who don't know what they're doing. But I've been really down since my old firm rejected me. I just don't get that attitude after all that I accomplished for them.

THERAPIST: Do you notice anything that happens or any thoughts or feelings you have just before the onset of your symptoms or a worsening of your problems?

MR. K: Mostly, I'm furious when I'm being mistreated. I can't believe these jerks don't recognize what I can accomplish for them. But sometimes I feel bad, like a loser. Or at least that's what I think new companies are going to think of me. I'm so worried about it that I haven't even applied for a new job. So, I'm kind of getting depressed.

THERAPIST: Are there any other problems you've been having?

MR. K: These work problems have really affected my relationship with my girlfriend. I lose my temper with her. And she's not really helping me deal with the stress. It sounds like you are feeling deeply hurt and angry about your skills not being recognized and this is triggering your depression. We'll explore what other factors in your life might contribute to these intense feeling to help you better manage them.

Relationship Problems

As noted, interpersonal problems have not been a focus of most psychodynamic psychotherapies. However, in problem-focused treatment, relationships are a central concern of the therapy and are addressed alongside other problems of the patient. Interpersonal problems can arise from many factors, including an inhibition about addressing problems with the other person, a sense of dependency on the other person, fears of disrupting the relationship, expressing aggression through rebellion or bullying, a lack of empathy for the other person's problems, and chronic conflicts that arise from a tendency to dramatize relationships or engage in sadomasochistic struggles.

Initial Evaluation of Relationship Problems

The dialogue that follows here revisits the case of Mr. F regarding his mention of relationship issues with his wife. It uses the guiding questions in Worksheet 2.8: Initial Evaluation of Relationship Problems (p. 56).

CASE EXAMPLE: MR. F'S RELATIONSHIP STRUGGLES

THERAPIST: What are the current problems you are struggling with in your relationships?

MR. F: The biggest problem is with my wife. She is constantly criticizing me about my working late and not doing enough with the kids. In actuality, I do a lot more than most fathers we know do. But somehow, it's not enough. But then she gets mad because we don't have more money. I get into big fights with her because I feel it's a no-win situation, and she doesn't seem to get it.

THERAPIST: Do you notice any triggers of these problems?

MR. F: The worst one is when I get home from work late. I try to get everything done and get home by 6, but a lot of times I end up staying late to complete everything. By the time I get home, she's in a big rage. Also, when she wants to buy something new for the house. I think she actually has kind of a shopping problem. Our financial problem really isn't that bad, but she's always wanting something new. This adds to the pressure.

THERAPIST: How long have you had these problems?

MR. F: We've always had some tension, but things got much worse with the new baby. Both the pressure I felt to work late and the amount of work at home shot up! I think that having a third kid was likely a mistake. Actually, I didn't really want another kid, but she insisted on it.

THERAPIST: How often do these problems occur?

MR. F: I guess it happens increasingly frequently. We fight a lot of the time. It's more like when *doesn't* it happen. There are stretches on weekends when I'm not busy where we can get along, and then we actually do great. But then, let's say on a Saturday afternoon, I say I have to work for an hour or so, she goes right back to being enraged. I just go work anyway. And that's when I might text with Sarah [the administrator with whom he has a flirtation] because I get so frustrated with my wife. At least that's fun and exciting. Or I may have a couple drinks.

Barriers to Recognizing Problems

Patients often have an inability or aversion to acknowledging or clarifying problems. Understanding these interfering factors is important for identifying both problems and associated intense negative feelings. Some of the more prevalent obstacles are denial, shame and guilt, and intrapsychic conflicts and defenses. Denial and shame often obscure substance use and other impulse-control problems. As noted above, patients with personality disorders often see these traits as part of themselves rather than as problems. Regarding interpersonal issues, patients often do not acknowledge their own contribution to difficulties, tending to blame the other person. Therapists help patients to both recognize their own contributions to problems and communicate more directly with others about problems.

Although it can take time for problems patients are embarrassed about to emerge in treatment, a simple query can sometimes help get a preliminary sense of some of these issues. Mr. F, for example, responded to his therapist by raising his conflicted feelings about the woman Sarah with whom he was having a flirtation.

THERAPIST: Are there problems or experiences that you're embarrassed to talk about?

MR. F: I don't really want to talk about my flirtation with Sarah. I mean nothing's happened, and I don't think I need to talk a lot about it. On the other hand, as I've been under more pressure and fighting with my wife, my urge to cross the line has increased. I know Susan isn't the type to put up with an affair. If she found out about it, things would probably be over between us.

Guilt, Shame, and Other Painful Feelings

The therapist should be alert and proceed tactfully with areas of difficulty that appear to make patients uncomfortable, as this can be an indicator of shame or guilt. A statement that many patients present with issues that are hard to talk about but are important to address can be helpful, along with a comment that the therapist will not be judgmental. Another way to get a sense of areas of shame is to ask patients directly about issues that trigger shame or guilt. Despite feeling embarrassed, some patients respond openly in the context of a general assessment, as they wish to talk about these painful issues. For example, the therapist picked up on Mr. H's distress as he talked about his family's reaction to his coming out, enabling him to describe some topics that were shameful to him.

THERAPIST: You seemed upset when you mentioned your family's reaction to your being gay. Can you say more about that?

MR. H: I still have some painful feelings about when I came out. It seemed to create a lot of trouble in my family. I feel they're still not fully accepting of me. Also, I had an incident in which I was molested when I was 15. I don't know how important it is, but I'm still not that comfortable talking about it. Maybe after we talk about some other things? But I do still feel ashamed about it and I still kind of blame myself.

The therapist responded by saying that he understood these experiences were very upsetting and felt they were important to talk more about when Mr. H felt more comfortable.

Another way that guilt or shame emerge is when therapists ask patients for more details about their problems, an often crucial means of better defining problems and their contributors. Patients may become hesitant to describe such details because they trigger painful feelings. Therapists can explain that understanding more details about these problems will help in gaining a better sense of how to relieve them. Therapists may sometimes note the patient's discomfort, as in, "You seem to be having a hard time providing me with more details. Are the questions bringing up some uncomfortable feelings?" Consider this dialogue, in which Ms. G, who struggled with anxiety and avoidant personality disorder, was discussing aspects of her social anxiety:

THERAPIST: Can you say more about what you actually experienced with others at the party?

MS. G: I just don't feel comfortable. I feel awkward.

THERAPIST: What types of situations trouble you?

MS. G: I hate it when I'm alone, wandering around at a party, and I can't find anyone to talk to. Or if people are together in a group. I don't want to try to break in.

THERAPIST: What would be the problem?

MS. G: What if they don't want me to be with them? Then I'll feel rejected. Or what if someone is mean?

THERAPIST: That would be upsetting. It sounds like you most worry about people excluding or rejecting you.

MS. G: I guess so. I haven't really thought of it that way.

THERAPIST: One of the questions we want to understand is why you're so worried about rejection. At parties, sometimes people are nice and sometimes not, and no one likes being excluded, but why does it trouble you so much?

MS. G: I'm not sure. That's a good question. But this is why I want to know who's going to be at the party. Or if my friend is going, I'll feel protected.

THERAPIST: So, it sounds like a friend would provide some sense of safety. You've told me that you have a number of friends and get along with others well. I think in general you overestimate the danger off rejection that you're in. And we want to understand why. Maybe something in your growing up.

MS. G: That's possible. I was attacked quite a bit by both my parents. I hadn't thought about that being connected.

This comment can now be followed up by exploring the patient's developmental history, as described in Chapter 3.

THERAPIST: Why don't you tell me something about those experiences?

Exploring Denial

Denial can function as a defense mechanism (see Chapter 5), a means of coping with internal states or external reality that feel intolerable or unacceptable. Although denial may be adaptive in certain circumstances when one is overwhelmed, persistent denial can lead to adverse outcomes with problems that must be addressed. For example, denial is common with substance misuse or abuse, as patients often deny or minimize their addictive behavior. Sometimes they will react quite negatively if the therapist presses them on these issues. So, while it is essential to inquire about possible addictive problems, the therapist should be sensitive in doing so. The therapist can also explore what makes the problem difficult to acknowledge.

CASE EXAMPLE: MR. F AND PROBLEM DRINKING

In the course of his evaluation of his overwork and anxiety, Mr. F revealed that he frequently drank alcohol on nights and weekends. He stated that this drinking helped him reduce work stress. He was cagey about the amount he drank. *The dialogue that follows here with Mr. F uses the guiding questions in Worksheet 2.9: Initial Evaluation of Addiction Problems (pp. 57–58).*

THERAPIST: Do you believe you have a drinking problem?

MR. F: I don't think I'm an alcoholic. I only end up having like three drinks a day. I know people who drink much more. And I can stop when I want. I've stopped for like a month a few weeks ago. But then I start again.

THERAPIST: Do you feel guilty about your drinking?

MR. F: I do feel guilty at times. I know I should stop entirely because it actually slows down my work, but I can't seem to do it. But I like getting the buzzed feeling. It gives me a big sense of relief from all the pressure, at least for a little while.

THERAPIST: Do you notice any triggers for your drinking?

MR. F: I feel so stressed out about work that I really need a few drinks in the evening when I get home to relax. And I'm still pretty anxious over the weekend, so I'll have a few drinks then, too.

THERAPIST: Have you tried to stop or cut back on your drinking? What happened with that?

MR. F: Yes, I did for about a month but then I got caught right back into the same pattern. I actually felt pretty good when I stopped. And guilty when I restarted. You'd think this would make it easier to try it again.

THERAPIST: What thoughts or feelings do you have about trying to cut back now?

MR. F: Well, I could say I'd be happy to try it but not right now because I have some get-togethers with friends coming up and we all drink together. I'm also worried that if I stop entirely, I'll get more anxious about work.

The Problem List

After identifying the patient's various problems, it is useful to construct a problem list. This list includes the problems the therapist and patient intend to target over the course of treatment. It can help maintain the focus in the treatment on the patient's problems, as is demonstrated throughout the course of this book. The list should not be rigidly adhered to, however, as new problems may emerge in the course of treatment that can be added to the list. The development of the list can enhance the therapeutic alliance, assuring that the problems the patient is concerned about are the focus of therapy. The problem list can also be used to assess the progress of treatment, in determining which problems are diminishing and which may be more persistent. In the latter case, a shift in strategy or therapeutic approach may be indicated. The therapist may create a mental list, share an actual list with the patient, or have patients develop their own list, which can be of value in maintaining focus and assessing progress on a given problem. For instance, the therapist created and presented the following problem list to Mr. F. He stated to him, "Here is my understanding of the problems we'll be working on together. Does this list make sense to you?"

1. Compulsive working
2. Generalized anxiety
3. Conflicts with your wife
4. Alcohol problems

Although he objected somewhat to his alcohol problems being noted, he did agree to consider that possibility and to leave it on the list.

RECOGNIZING THAT PROBLEMS HAVE MEANINGS AND FUNCTIONS

In the process of identifying problems, the PrFPP therapist communicates that they represent usually unconscious efforts to solve certain difficulties, which are often maladaptive. Defining problems and exploring the associated context and feelings provide information that is useful in understanding these meanings. For example, somatic symptoms are identified as an attempt to manage psychological and emotional states rather than as a bodily problem. Focus on the body can be a defense against painful conflicted feelings and fantasies, or it can symbolize an intrapsychic conflict, often involving dependency or aggression. For example, the therapist noted how Ms. I focused on her body when she had increased conflicts with her friends and that these symptoms seemed to be part of an effort to manage her very intense feelings of anger, hurt, and rejection. Her experience that her body was out of control (e.g., a brain tumor) could be linked to a fear that her emotions were out of control. The therapist indicates that understanding these meanings enables a means of addressing contributors to problems. Establishing that symptoms, behaviors, personality issues, and relationship difficulties have meanings and functions is a core part of PrFPP.

IDENTIFYING AND ADDRESSING THE IMPACT OF CULTURAL FACTORS

Recognizing and exploring the role of cultural factors is essential in the identification and treatment of problems. Patients' cultural backgrounds strongly influence both the nature and perception of their difficulties and which problems they feel safe or unsafe discussing. Additionally, some subcultures are more likely to experience certain forms of trauma, such as those that result from the impact of institutionalized racism and poverty. If such factors are not taken into account, it could interfere with the alliance with certain patients and their sense of safety in revealing problems. Examples that arose in the cases presented in this chapter included Ms. I, whose experiences of racism emerged as important contributors to her conflicted anger and anxiety. She recalled warnings from her mother to be deferential to White people, even if mistreated. In the case of Mr. H, the culture of the country he was from was very hostile toward homosexuality. In addition to his family, this attitude added to his internalized negative feelings about being gay.

RECOGNIZING RELEVANT DYNAMICS

Defining underlying dynamics that contribute to various problems is a key aspect of PrFPP. Preliminary dynamic information often emerges and can be identified when creating a problem list. In an early session, for example, the therapist noted that Mr. A tended to take back angry comments or feel guilty after expressing anger. In the course of his treatment, the therapist identified how conflicts about angry feelings and fantasies contributed to various problems, including symptoms (anxiety/panic), behavioral problems (passive–aggressive behavior with his husband, as he was unable to express anger directly), personality difficulties (unassertiveness), and relationship issues (e.g., difficulty addressing his needs and frustrations with his husband). In addition, developmental contributors often begin to emerge, as with Ms. G's recognition that criticism from her family while growing up contributed to her fears.

A framework for identifying and addressing dynamics is described in Chapters 3 through 7, which focus on these topics.

> **QUESTIONS AND IDEAS TO THINK ABOUT**
>
> 1. With a new patient or one you are currently working with, try identifying and dividing the patient's problems into a list, considering symptoms, personality issues, behavioral difficulties, and relationship problems. How does this affect your thinking and approach to the patient?
> 2. Once you have a problem list, explore what might contribute to exacerbation or relief of these problems. Do you notice any patterns or triggers? Does this information suggest any options for interventions that were not evident before?

HANDOUT 2.1

Introduction to the Treatment

In this treatment, we will be working to understand the symptoms and problems you have and what contributes to them, enabling you to better recognize and address them. These problems include symptoms, behavioral issues, and relationship difficulties. Problems are usually found to have developed or worsen in certain situations or become triggered by certain thoughts or feelings. Factors from your childhood and past often contribute to the development of problems. Exploring these contributing factors will improve your capacity to intervene with them. Your therapist will work with you to identify the specific problems you have in language that makes sense to you and to make a list of these problems. Although it may seem self-evident what problems you suffer from, sometimes people are not aware of certain problems they have; the therapist will help you to identify these. Additionally, people may struggle with or deny problems they feel guilty and ashamed about but need help with, which the therapist will explore in a nonjudgmental manner.

From *Skills Training in Psychodynamic Psychotherapy*, by Fredric N. Busch. Copyright © 2026 The Guilford Press. Permission to photocopy this handout, or to download and print additional copies (*www.guilford.com/busch-forms*), is granted to purchasers of this book for personal use or use with clients; see copyright page for details.

WORKSHEET 2.1

Initial Identification of Problems

These questions will help you and your therapist identify and understand any problems you may be having and collect your thoughts about things that may trigger these problems. These questions are also intended to help you become more alert to the thoughts, feelings, and circumstances associated with your problems to help you and your therapist better address them.

How would you describe the main concerns or problems that brought you in for therapy?

How severe are these problems? How much are they disrupting your life?

Do you believe there are triggers of these problems? If so, what might they be?

(continued)

From *Skills Training in Psychodynamic Psychotherapy*, by Fredric N. Busch. Copyright © 2026 The Guilford Press. Permission to photocopy this worksheet, or to download and print additional copies (*www.guilford.com/busch-forms*), is granted to purchasers of this book for personal use or use with clients; see copyright page for details.

Initial Identification of Problems *(page 2 of 2)*

What was going on in your life when you started having these problems? What were the various stresses in your life at that time? Are they still present?

Do you notice anything that happens or any thoughts or feelings you have just before the onset of your symptoms or a worsening of your problems?

Are there any other problems you've been having?

WORKSHEET 2.2

Initial Evaluation of Anxiety

These questions will help you and your therapist gather information about any anxiety you may be feeling and what circumstances trigger or worsen your anxiety.

Have you been experiencing anxiety?

How severe has it been?

How frequently do you experience anxiety? Do you feel it much of the time or only occasionally?

(continued)

From *Skills Training in Psychodynamic Psychotherapy*, by Fredric N. Busch. Copyright © 2026 The Guilford Press. Permission to photocopy this worksheet, or to download and print additional copies (*www.guilford.com/busch-forms*), is granted to purchasers of this book for personal use or use with clients; see copyright page for details.

Initial Evaluation of Anxiety *(page 2 of 2)*

What kinds of circumstances trigger your anxiety?

What kinds of thoughts accompany your anxiety? Can you describe them?

When did your anxiety start? What was going on in your life at that time?

Do you have panic attacks (episodes of severe anxiety accompanied by symptoms such as chest pain, shortness of breath, palpitations, catastrophic feelings of doom)? Do you notice any particular circumstances or thoughts and feelings that trigger your panic episodes?

WORKSHEET 2.3

Initial Evaluation of Depression

These questions will help you and your therapist gather information about any feelings of depression you may be experiencing, as well as what kinds of circumstances, thoughts, and feelings might trigger or worsen your depression.

Have you ever felt down or depressed?

How intense has your depression been?

Can you describe your symptoms?

(continued)

From *Skills Training in Psychodynamic Psychotherapy*, by Fredric N. Busch. Copyright © 2026 The Guilford Press. Permission to photocopy this worksheet, or to download and print additional copies (*www.guilford.com/busch-forms*), is granted to purchasers of this book for personal use or use with clients; see copyright page for details.

Initial Evaluation of Depression *(page 2 of 2)*

Have you noticed any triggers of your symptoms?

What kinds of thoughts and feelings do you have when you're down?

Do you get self-critical?

Are there any other issues you believe are contributing to your depression?

WORKSHEET 2.4
Initial Evaluation of Somatic Symptoms

These questions will help you and your therapist gather information about any bodily symptoms you may be experiencing and your concerns about them. These questions can also help you think about any circumstances, thoughts, or feelings that may be triggering your symptoms.

Do you have any concerns or worries about your body? If so, can you describe them?

How long have you had these worries?

What was going on in your life when these worries started? Any particular stresses?

(continued)

From *Skills Training in Psychodynamic Psychotherapy*, by Fredric N. Busch. Copyright © 2026 The Guilford Press. Permission to photocopy this worksheet, or to download and print additional copies (www.guilford.com/busch-forms), is granted to purchasers of this book for personal use or use with clients; see copyright page for details.

Initial Evaluation of Somatic Symptoms *(page 2 of 2)*

Have these stresses caused you significant distress?

Have you had fears like this before? Were any stresses associated with those fears?

Have you been to the doctor about this problem or other concerns about your health? What have the doctors said?

WORKSHEET 2.5

Initial Evaluation of Inhibited Behaviors

These questions will help you and your therapist identify behaviors that you want to engage in but feel inhibited from doing. These questions may also help you begin to consider what causes these inhibitions to better address them in therapy.

Are there behaviors you want to engage in but feel inhibited from doing?

Can you describe those behaviors?

Can you describe what inhibits you from doing them?

(continued)

From *Skills Training in Psychodynamic Psychotherapy*, by Fredric N. Busch. Copyright © 2026 The Guilford Press. Permission to photocopy this worksheet, or to download and print additional copies (*www.guilford.com/busch-forms*), is granted to purchasers of this book for personal use or use with clients; see copyright page for details.

Initial Evaluation of Inhibited Behaviors *(page 2 of 2)*

Are there certain circumstances in which you feel more inhibitions about these behaviors? Can you describe them?

When did these inhibitions start? Were there any particular stresses in your life at that time?

WORKSHEET 2.6

Initial Evaluation of Behaviors That Are Difficult to Control

These questions will help you and your therapist gather information about behaviors you have trouble controlling (impulses). This information will also help you and your therapist think about triggers of these behaviors to help you better manage them.

Do you have trouble controlling certain behaviors or impulses? Sexual wishes? Temper? Alcohol or drugs? Shopping?

Do you notice any triggers for these behaviors?

When did these problems start? Were there any particular stresses in your life at that time?

(continued)

From *Skills Training in Psychodynamic Psychotherapy*, by Fredric N. Busch. Copyright © 2026 The Guilford Press. Permission to photocopy this worksheet, or to download and print additional copies (www.guilford.com/busch-forms), is granted to purchasers of this book for personal use or use with clients; see copyright page for details.

Initial Evaluation of Behaviors That Are Difficult to Control *(page 2 of 2)*

Do you feel guilty about these behaviors?

What are the consequences of these behaviors?

Have you tried to get control over these behaviors?

WORKSHEET 2.7

Initial Evaluation of Avoidant Tendencies

These questions will help you and your therapist gather information about tendencies to avoid situations based on your anxiety.

Does your anxiety lead you to avoid certain situations?

How long have you had these avoidance problems?

Are you aware of triggers of this avoidance or of situations that make it worse?

What kinds of thoughts precede or accompany your fears and avoidance?

From *Skills Training in Psychodynamic Psychotherapy*, by Fredric N. Busch. Copyright © 2026 The Guilford Press. Permission to photocopy this worksheet, or to download and print additional copies (*www.guilford.com/busch-forms*), is granted to purchasers of this book for personal use or use with clients; see copyright page for details.

WORKSHEET 2.8

Initial Evaluation of Relationship Problems

These questions will help you and your therapist gather information about any relationship problems you may be having. This information will also help identify ways of addressing these problems.

What are the current problems you are struggling with in your relationships?

Do you notice any triggers of these problems?

How long have you had these problems?

How often do these problems occur?

From *Skills Training in Psychodynamic Psychotherapy*, by Fredric N. Busch. Copyright © 2026 The Guilford Press. Permission to photocopy this worksheet, or to download and print additional copies (*www.guilford.com/busch-forms*), is granted to purchasers of this book for personal use or use with clients; see copyright page for details.

WORKSHEET 2.9

Initial Evaluation of Addiction Problems

These questions will help you and your therapist gather information about any substance misuse or abuse that can accompany or contribute to various problems. This worksheet focuses on alcohol, but any substance can be substituted. It is also of value for identifying triggers of your use of substances that can be targeted in treatment.

Do you believe you have a drinking problem?

Do you feel guilty about your drinking?

Do you notice any triggers of your drinking?

(continued)

From *Skills Training in Psychodynamic Psychotherapy*, by Fredric N. Busch. Copyright © 2026 The Guilford Press. Permission to photocopy this worksheet, or to download and print additional copies (www.guilford.com/busch-forms), is granted to purchasers of this book for personal use or use with clients; see copyright page for details.

Initial Evaluation of Addiction Problems *(page 2 of 2)*

Have you tried to stop or cut back on your drinking? What happened with that?

What thoughts or feelings do you have about trying to cut back now?

CHAPTER 3

Identifying and Addressing the Situations, Emotions, Thoughts, and Developmental Factors Contributing to Problems

Self-observation is an essential tool in examining factors contributing to problems and developing interventions to address them, as discussed in Chapter 2. The therapist works to enhance the patients' self-observational capacities, beginning with the identification of problems and continuing in efforts to explore the surrounding context, mental states, and emotions. The therapist helps patients clarify their experiences at the time problems developed, as well as recent triggers that worsen problems. A diary in which patients can record the context, thoughts, and feelings surrounding problems, described below, further promotes the development of this skill (Busch, 2018). Identifying these factors will aid patients in feeling more control over their issues and help them recognize and manage emotional and cognitive triggers.

Self-observational skills also help to develop a "staging area" for addressing problems or intervening with them. Many patients, for example, report that impulsive behaviors occur so rapidly that they do not have an opportunity to even consider stopping them. Additionally, inhibitions of behaviors tend to occur reflexively, and patients often do not think about what leads to these inhibitions. Furthermore, problems perform an important psychic function for the patient, sometimes creating a resistance to exploring these factors. For instance, agoraphobic symptoms can protect a patient from fears of separation and anger. These contributing conflicts and defenses are addressed further in Chapter 5. The development of a "staging area" allows the patient an opportunity to step back from various problems, identify their sources, and consider ways to address them. In this chapter, examples are given on how to use diaries and worksheets to improve self-observational skills and intervene with various problems.

Three metaphors are useful for describing the process of self-observation, identifying contributors to problems, and determining interventions. **Building a scaffold** allows closer observation of and access to a structure, enabling repair, just as self-observation aids in identifying problems and their contributors. The elaboration of context, emotions, thoughts, and dynamic factors as viewed from a "scaffold" provides a series of intervention points for addressing problems. Self-observation can be compared to **reviewing a video** of the thoughts, feelings, and situations that precede or surround certain problems. Thus, patients can be asked to describe, as best they can, the events, mental states, and behaviors that occur during that time, as if they were reviewing a video. Analyzing the information from the "video" can help derive and test new intervention strategies. Viewing problems as **whirlpools** can express the patient's feelings of lack of control and being caught by problems. If the individual does not recognize the problem, the therapist helps identify that the patient is in a whirlpool and works to clarify its nature. Therapist and patient then undertake efforts to understand the currents (e.g., stressors, emotions, thoughts, behaviors, conflicts, and defenses) that contribute to the whirlpool and its intensity and develop strategies to get out (see Handout 3.1, p. 75).

MONITORING CIRCUMSTANCES, THOUGHTS, FEELINGS, AND REACTIONS SURROUNDING PROBLEMS

Patients can be given a diary/worksheet to better monitor their problems and relevant triggers. (A blank diary page, Worksheet 3.1: Monitoring Circumstances, Thoughts, Feelings, and Reactions Surrounding Problems (p. 76), as well as all other worksheets in this chapter, is available online at *www.guilford.com/busch-forms*.) Patients should be encouraged to make a notation in their diary whenever they observe the onset of worsening of a problem. Categories (placed in columns) include circumstances, thoughts, feelings, and reactions. Keeping such a log of these experiences will aid patients in developing the capacity to attend to the problems that are troubling them and begin to define the stressors, emotions, and thoughts that contribute to them. Ms. L (in the case that follows) filled out a diary, which was helpful for her and her therapist to connect her problems and triggers and work on approaching these situations differently.

CASE EXAMPLE: MS. L

Ms. L, a 70-year-old Black retiree struggling with depression and anxiety, completed a diary as she monitored what triggered or worsened her symptoms (see Figure 3.1).

After reviewing Ms. L's log, the therapist asked for more specifics about her experiences and observations surrounding the exacerbation of the problems that occurred with her aunt:

THERAPIST: Had you been aware that your interactions with your aunt triggered your symptoms?

MS. L: I knew about the tensions between us, but I hadn't noticed that my guilt and anxiety got worse after our fights until I began filling out the diary. I also hadn't recognized how demeaning her comments were about me. I usually ended up stewing about her remarks, but I figured I was just being too sensitive.

THERAPIST: Can you tell me more details about the thoughts, feelings, and behaviors you mentioned in the diary? Maybe you can describe it as if you were reviewing a video of what happened as you experienced this problem with her.

MS. L: I quickly realized that I was being insulted and got mad. And instead of just stewing, I blurted out that she was a nasty person who was always being judgmental. She became quiet and looked hurt. Then I felt guilty because I know she's old, and this is just the way she is. That's when I started feeling more down and anxious that I had somehow pushed her away or hurt her. After the incident, I felt kind of stuck and preoccupied. I went back and forth between feeling mad and like I should say something and feel guilty about how I reacted.

Below is a diary to help monitor your problems and relevant triggers. Make a notation in your diary whenever you note the onset or worsening of a problem. Keeping such a log of these experiences will aid you in developing the capacity to attend to the problems that are troubling you and begin to define the stressors, emotions, and thoughts that contribute to them.

Date and Time	Circumstances Describe what was happening at that time.	Thoughts	Feelings	Reactions Describe how you reacted.
Saturday, February 15	I had a fight with my aunt. She insulted me by saying, "I was always having technical problems" in a disdainful way when I was talking about difficulties I was having with my computer.	It wasn't true what she said. I have tech problems on occasion, but so do many other people. I was thinking that she just wants to feel superior.	I got furious with her.	I said some mean things to my aunt, but then I felt guilty and down.

FIGURE 3.1. Diary entry for Ms. L: Monitoring Circumstances, Thoughts, Feelings, and Reactions Surrounding Problems.

After the therapist heard more about this incident, he commented on the anger, depression, and guilt it caused:

THERAPIST: I think it's understandable that you would react angrily to your aunt's critical comments, so we need to understand why it makes you feel so guilty. We can also discuss ways to express your anger differently. Perhaps you could say something like "Wow that comment was kind of harsh" instead of something negative about her.

MS. L: Those are good suggestions. Now that I've become more aware of her attacks on me, I think I can get a jump start in dealing with them. But I get furious very quickly and worry I'll just say something hurtful.

As in the above exchange, therapists using PrFPP may sometimes suggest alternative behaviors for the patient to consider that emerge from exploring contributors to problems (Busch, 2018).

Linking

This therapeutic technique connects patients' problems to particular feelings, thoughts, circumstances, representations of self and others, and developmental experiences. Linking also can help to make somatic symptoms meaningful to a patient by connecting their bodily experiences with particular mental states and situational triggers. Making such connections plays an important role in helping patients identify contributors to the development and persistence of their problems. Initially, linkages involve particular emotions, stressors, and thoughts associated with a patient's problem. From there, aspects of developmental history, self and other representations, and conflicts can also be connected, further elaborating the psychodynamic formulation.

The cases described below demonstrate the process of making early linkages, such as connecting Mr. M's receiving negative news about his business to his panic, sense of catastrophe, and feelings of failure. Further information about Mr. M presented later in the chapter connects his presenting problems to his developmental history.

CASE EXAMPLE: MR. M

Mr. M was a 62-year-old White married businessman with a history of a past business failure, but his current company had been successful for many years. He presented with anxious and depressive symptoms, including panic attacks. These symptoms arose as he experienced a recent downturn in his business, although he acknowledged that, overall, it was doing well. In Figure 3.2 are Mr. M's responses to his diary monitoring circumstances, thoughts, feelings, and behavior.

Below is a diary to help monitor your problems and relevant triggers. Make a notation in your diary whenever you note the onset or worsening of a problem. Keeping such a log of these experiences will aid you in developing the capacity to attend to the problems that are troubling you and begin to define the stressors, emotions, and thoughts that contribute to them.

Date	Circumstances Describe what was happening at that time.	Thoughts	Feelings	Reactions Describe how you reacted.
Tuesday, February 25	I didn't get a payment we expected yesterday, and I realized we might end up operating at a loss this month.	I suddenly had the thought that my business was going to completely collapse. Then I'd be a failure. And then I started worrying that it's because I'm too old. Maybe I just don't have what it takes anymore.	I went into a panic. I felt like things were catastrophic. My heart started beating really rapidly, and my body felt very tense. I was worried I might have been having a heart attack.	I was so anxious I couldn't go to sleep. I stayed up most of the night thinking about how I might get some new initiatives going, but I wasn't really getting much done.

FIGURE 3.2. Diary entry for Mr. M: Monitoring Circumstances, Thoughts, Feelings, and Reactions Surrounding Problems.

The therapist explored Mr. M's panic attacks further, using the guiding questions from Worksheet 3.2: Assessing Triggers and Content of Panic Attacks (p. 77).

THERAPIST: What kinds of feelings or experiences did you notice preceded your panic?

MR. M: I'm always worried that my business is on the verge of falling apart. Anytime there's a slowdown, I start to panic, and I think it's all over.

THERAPIST: Can you give me the details of a specific trigger?

MR. M: The incident I described in my diary was a bad month, but even not getting a payment for one day or a bad week can lead me to panic. And somehow, it's hard for me to think at that point how the business is actually doing pretty well overall.

THERAPIST: What thoughts and fears accompanied your panic?

MR. M: Once I start panicking, my thoughts get increasingly dire. First, that the business is going to fall apart entirely. Next, that I'm a failure or that I'm having a heart attack. I hadn't realized how quickly it all happened.

THERAPIST: Do you have a sense of other problems or tensions in your life that may contribute to these fears?

MR. M: I'm really worried about getting older and that I won't be able to manage the business in the same way. Then what would I do?

The therapist, after reviewing Mr. M's diary entry above, made the following intervention:

THERAPIST: From what you've said and the note in your diary this week, it seems clear that some of the triggers of your panic are minor downturns in your business. But these downturns aren't really affecting its overall success. We need to try to understand what contributes to this whirlpool feeling of everything falling apart. And we also need to look at this sense of being a failure.

MR. M: I still think it's very scary. A whirlpool is a good way of putting it because I feel completely out of control and fear that the business will collapse. Maybe it has to do with my past business failure. And the failure feelings remind me of something my dad often said, that I wouldn't amount to anything. I'd like to talk more about that.

THERAPIST: Yes, those connections to your past experiences will be helpful in understanding and addressing your panic because your business is not at risk of falling apart now.

CASE EXAMPLE: MS. J

Ms. J, described in Chapter 2 and who struggled with compulsive shopping, made some observations in her diary when she experienced an impulse to shop (see Figure 3.3).

She then responded to a question from her therapist that asked her to summarize what she learned from her diary:

THERAPIST: What did you observe about the circumstances, feelings, and thoughts that preceded acting on your impulses.

MS. J: I realized that my shopping spree occurred just after I had a fight with my husband, or I felt dissed at work. I guess I'm really mad and feel deprived, and shopping makes me feel better. I feel like I'm being treated unfairly at home and work, like I'm not getting the positive feedback or regard I should get.

THERAPIST: I think it's important that we understand the intensity of your feelings of being deprived and angry because it seems like you attempt to relieve them by buying things, but I'm not sure that ultimately helps.

MS. J: It's true because I just end up having these feelings again. But I've never really stopped and thought about them.

Below is a diary to help monitor your problems and relevant triggers. Make a notation in your diary whenever you note the onset or worsening of a problem. Keeping such a log of these experiences will aid you in developing the capacity to attend to the problems that are troubling you and begin to define the stressors, emotions, and thoughts that contribute to them.

Date	Circumstances Describe what was happening at that time.	Thoughts	Feelings	Reactions Describe how you reacted.
Wednesday, February 5	I had a fight with my husband about him always being so negative. I'd also had a bad day at work. I'm just not getting the recognition I deserve for what I contribute.	I had the thought that I'm really sick of my husband. He's such a downer, and so is work. And then I thought of going shopping. That would at least perk me up a bit.	I was furious at him. And I felt hurt and angry about the situation at work.	I went right to the store and started shopping. I didn't even worry about how much things cost or what the credit card bill would look like.

FIGURE 3.3. Diary entry for Ms. J: Monitoring Circumstances, Thoughts, Feelings, and Reactions Surrounding Problems.

USING DIARIES AND WORKSHEETS TO ADDRESS IMPULSIVE BEHAVIORS AND INHIBITIONS

In addition to identifying contributors to problems and symptoms as described previously, diaries regarding context, emotions, and thoughts are also important in developing and attempting interventions to make changes in problematic behaviors.

The following guided questions are used to help patients explore what it would feel like to not act on an impulsive behavior. Use Worksheet 3.3: Exploring Not Acting on an Impulsive Behavior (pp. 78–79) with these questions.

Mr. F, described in Chapter 2, responded to these questions about his impulse to take on new clients, even when he was too busy, in the following way:

THERAPIST: If you imagine not acting on the impulse to behave in this way, what do you think will happen or that you'll experience?

MR. F: I don't know. First, I think I owe it to new clients to take them on because I think I'm really good at the job and they need help. But also, if I don't take on the client, I'm worried that I'll feel really bad about myself and about losing the money.

THERAPIST: Are you certain that you'll have a negative reaction?

MR. F: I can't really be sure about it because I've never really tried it, but I'm pretty sure that's how I will feel because I get this feeling even when I just think about it.

THERAPIST: How do you feel when you've acted on the impulse?

MR. F: I feel terrible because I know it's not good for me, and my wife gets very upset. But I can't really stop myself from doing it.

THERAPIST: Let's have you try holding off acting on the impulse as a test to see what will happen. Then we can discuss what you experienced when you delay the behavior.

Following this session, Mr. F was able to delay accepting one of his new referrals to test out this experience. If the patient is unable to take this step, then the therapist works further on contributors to the behavior and ways of holding off on the impulsive behavior. This therapeutic exchange explored his experience further (see a continuation of Worksheet 3.3: Exploring Not Acting on an Impulsive Behavior [pp. 78–79]):

THERAPIST: What thoughts and feelings did you have when you held off acting on the impulse?

MR. F: I felt guilty at first when I thought about not taking on the client. Kind of this lack of value. Or like I'm letting somebody down. But then I also felt potential relief, like reduced pressure from work and maybe more time with my family. Then I decided I just better take the client.

THERAPIST: Are you willing to try it again?

MR. F: It's scary. I don't know how well I would handle it. I mean maybe I'll feel more of the relief. Maybe I'll feel more of the bad feelings.

The therapist then explored this experience further:

THERAPIST: So, I think it was good that you held off taking the client for a period. I think we want to understand more about the feelings you described. I know you referred to a lack of value and letting someone down. Those both seem painful and important.

MR. F: I felt kind of worthless. Like if I'm not busy all the time, I don't have any value. It's a terrible feeling. I know you've mentioned that maybe this is related to my father being demanding, but I'm not sure.

THERAPIST: That makes sense, and I think we need to explore these thoughts and feelings further because it's important to understand how you could possibly feel of no value given the efforts that you make for your business and family. And what about letting others down?

MR. F: I know it doesn't make sense, but I feel like my business will fall apart and I won't be able to support my wife and family. Then I'll really feel like a failure.

THERAPIST: This indicates why it's important for you to try to hold off, not only because you're pushing yourself to work in a way that creates stress for you and your family, but you're also trying to push away feelings and thoughts that don't make rational sense and are important to understand.

MR. F: I see what you're saying because I also felt that sense of relief.

Therapists can use a similar approach and guiding questions to address inhibited behaviors. (See Worksheet 3.4: Exploring Enacting an Inhibited Behavior [pp. 80–81].) For example, in the case of Mr. A, the therapist worked with him to be more assertive in expressing his frustration with his husband. They explored what came to mind when he considered addressing one of their issues (wanting Joseph to give him less advice) and identified that Mr. A had fears of being rejected or punished. They discussed what he might say to Joseph in this context that might be helpful rather than provoke irritation. They talked about how it felt important to address these difficulties, even if Joseph responded angrily. Ultimately, Mr. A was able to bring up his feelings of being intruded upon, and his husband, somewhat to Mr. A's surprise, was quite responsive. The therapist worked with this positive result to further address Mr. A's fears of assertion.

EXPLORING THE RELEVANCE OF DEVELOPMENTAL EXPERIENCES TO CURRENT PROBLEMS

The psychodynamic therapist works to identify the relevance of the patient's history to current problems. As noted in Chapter 1, early life experiences play a key role in the development and content of self and other representations, the nature and intensity of the patient's intrapsychic conflicts, and the patient's capability for mentalization and symbolization. The therapist can explore the patient's early experiences with a guided interview.

Understanding how developmental factors contribute to current difficulties helps therapists and patients understand the source of patients' problems and better manage them. An important link to past events is found not only in the nature of the problems, but the circumstances, feelings, and thoughts surrounding them. As the patient's problems and context are identified and the developmental history is obtained, therapist and patient can begin to identify these links.

The case of Mr. M illustrates the use of the guiding questions in Worksheet 3.5: Exploring Developmental History (pp. 82–84) to identify relevant developmental factors.

CASE EXAMPLE: MR. M

Mr. M, the 62-year-old married businessman described earlier, presented for evaluation of depression, anxiety, and panic attacks associated with fears of his business failing, associated with a view of himself as being "bad." His anxiety and self-criticisms persisted despite his business remaining profitable and his finances stable. He did have a business failure many years previously but rebuilt the business by shifting his focus. He was also critical of his children's inability to be financially independent, and felt pressure to keep working to help support them. He would become preoccupied with fears of dying, which were later found to be associated with being abandoned or punished.

Mr. M stated that his parents viewed him as a "bad kid." However, he reported that he rarely got into trouble outside of his home and that he believed his parents' perception was unfair. Exploration suggested that his "badness" related to his parents' attitude toward his struggle with limits (e.g., defying them about curfews, use of the car), a tendency that he felt contributed subsequently to his business successes. Nevertheless, this sense of being bad persisted and worsened when he struggled more with business, as he recalled his parents saying, "You won't amount to anything." He believed his problems began with the birth of his brother at age 4, feeling ignored by his parents. His brother was always perceived as "the good one," being much more compliant. He subsequently took satisfaction in being more successful than his brother, although he experienced some guilt about this. He described one supportive figure in his early life, his grandmother, with whom he experienced a sense of warmth that he felt was missing in his parents.

The therapist explored Mr. M's developmental history using the guiding questions from Worksheet 3.5 (pp. 82–84):

THERAPIST: Can you describe your parents? What were they like?

MR. M: They were hardworking people. My father owned a store. They weren't particularly mean but didn't really know much about dealing with feelings. I guess I just felt alone.

THERAPIST: Can you describe your parents' attitudes and behavior toward you? Did you consider your early environment abusive or neglectful in any way?

MR. M: Everything was okay until my brother came along when I was 4. I felt my parents loved him more. And somehow, I was just seen as "bad," always causing trouble. But I don't think I was really bad. Probably normal kid things. I did take the car for a drive at age 12. Things like that.

THERAPIST: How were anxiety and separations managed in the family?

MR. M: I was worried because I felt I was always going to be in trouble. But I don't remember any problems with separation. In fact, I ran away from home when I was 8, but my parents found me pretty quickly.

THERAPIST: How was anger managed in the family?

MR. M: I felt like my parents were always angry at me. I got mad at them, but that just got them angrier. They probably just saw it as an example of my being bad.

THERAPIST: Did your parents fight? How much? About what?

MR. M: They didn't fight that much. At least not that I was aware of.

THERAPIST: What were your siblings like? What were your experiences with your siblings?

MR. M: My brother was probably fine, but I was always angry toward him and jealous of the attention that he got. We're not really close now.

THERAPIST: Were there other significant caregivers in your early life (e.g., grandparents, nanny)?

MR. M: There was my grandmother. I felt she understood me and didn't see me in the same way. But she actually spoke very little English. She was kind of a warm presence.

THERAPIST: What was the environment you grew up in like (cultural, religious, financial, etc.)?

MR. M: It was a middle-class Jewish family. My parents were okay financially. But we lived in a part of the city I thought of as a backwater. I always wanted out.

THERAPIST: Did you experience any major losses, injuries growing up?

MR. M: Not really. My grandmother died when I was 14. I was sad, but I just felt she was kind of old.

THERAPIST: Did you have any experiences you would consider traumatic growing up?

MR. M: I guess if you think of always being seen as bad as traumatic. I just know it really affected me. It stayed with me.

Mr. M also made an entry in his diary (see Figure 3.4).

In examining the diaries and the contexts of resurgences of symptoms, Mr. M and his therapist identified that his fears and depressive feelings were triggered by reminders of his past business failure but were further exacerbated when he felt rejected or alone. For instance, the therapist and he were able to recognize that he became more frightened about his business when his wife was away. Using this information, the therapist made a developmental interpretation, connecting his past experiences to his current problems. He suggested that Mr. M felt rejected or emotionally abandoned by his parents from viewing him as "bad" and in part accepted his parents' critical view. Although he became angry at them for their harsh judgment, he did not feel safe with these feelings and directed them inward with self-criticism. Mr. M felt this perspective helped him better understand the surge in his negative feelings.

Below is a diary to help monitor your problems and relevant triggers. Make a notation in your diary whenever you note the onset or worsening of a problem. Keeping such a log of these experiences will aid you in developing the capacity to attend to the problems that are troubling you and begin to define the stressors, emotions, and thoughts that contribute to them.

Date	Circumstances Describe what was happening at that time.	Thoughts	Feelings	Reactions Describe how you reacted.
Friday, February 7	I noticed that my anxiety about business got worse when I was feeling alone when my wife went on a trip. Also, around the same time, I found out my earnings were down the prior month.	I thought that I had failed and that I was a bad person. And I felt like my business was falling apart, even though these were only minor blips. Somehow, I started focusing on my past business failures.	I felt intense anxiety about failing in my business and that it had something to do with my being a bad person.	I felt helpless and stuck. I couldn't figure out what to do.

FIGURE 3.4. Diary entry for Mr. M: Monitoring Circumstances, Thoughts, Feelings, and Reactions Surrounding Problems..

An additional example of the impact of his early history emerged within the transference when the therapist went on vacation, as Mr. M reported that he felt like "a failure, bad, I've done something wrong. I'm in trouble and frightened about my finances. I'm back in the whirlpool." He continued to use the term "whirlpool" to refer to his state of feeling bad and catastrophically fearful about his business. Another "current" contributing to the whirlpool was that he just learned that a prior client had switched to a competitor, leaving Mr. M feeling angry and rejected, though that prior client had not been a major source of income.

In exploring the resurgence of symptoms, Mr. M described hurt and anger at both his client and the therapist. He linked it to his brother getting the attention for being good, while he was seen as the bad one.

MR. M: I felt very alone when this client went to my competitor. Your being away didn't help.

THERAPIST: I understand that. We've also recognized that, when you feel alone or rejected, you believe you're being punished for being bad.

MR. M: I think that makes sense. My parents didn't understand what was going on with me emotionally. And when they punished me, they barely talked to me. Now that I think about it, my wife was also away when this happened.

THERAPIST: So, that further explains why you felt so abandoned and punished.

MR. M: Somehow this brought to mind my business collapsing 30 years ago. It was so scary because I had to borrow money to keep going. I felt lonely, anxious, and depressed. I had to get help from a psychiatrist at that time also.

THERAPIST: That sounds like a traumatic experience that likely contributes to your current fears. But you're not in danger financially now.

MR. M: And my client choosing a competitor reminded me of the loss when my brother came on the scene. That probably led me to feel more threatened.

THERAPIST: I think that's a very important connection that you're making.

MR. M: But how do I keep this in mind when I'm feeling panicky?

THERAPIST: It might help to think of it as building a scaffold, a way to step back and consider your problems from a different perspective, using what you've learned about them. For example, you can challenge your fears with your awareness of how your business is doing okay and that your fears actually come from experiences in your past.

MR. M: That's a good idea. I'll try that because it's hard to keep that in mind when I get anxious.

Mr. M's question about how to make changes when feelings and fears appear overwhelming is a common one. The analogy of a scaffold, or staging area, can provide patients with concrete ways of thinking about a place in their mind from which they can challenge their symptoms and problems.

Identifying the contexts of Mr. M's catastrophic fears furthered an understanding of contributing dynamic factors, enabling links to his developmental history and the transference. The therapist worked with the patient's equating separation with rejection and his sense of being bad, which were displaced to anxiety about his finances. This formulation helped Mr. M recognize that the dangers he experienced derived from emotional and developmental factors rather than the current reality. Being able to address his fears of abandonment and rejection directly with the therapist further helped relieve his anxieties.

CASE EXAMPLE: MS. N'S PANIC

Ms. N, a 27-year-old Latina nurse, quickly gained a sense of the link between current life stressors, developmental experiences, and her recent surge of anxiety and panic. She recognized that her panic attacks began shortly after the sudden death of one of her patients. She acknowledged that she was not particularly close to the patient and had seen other patients die, but the death struck her as "unfair" because the patient was young and improving. Although this event was the immediate precipitant, further exploration revealed that she was anxious and frustrated with her work and her boyfriend. At her job, she felt fearful and pressured to keep up with her duties and believed she was underpaid, which she also found to be unfair. Additionally, she found her boyfriend, with whom she had recently broken up, to be "cold and callous" and she was having intense episodes or anxiety about the possibility of breaking up with him.

THERAPIST: Tell me about the problems with your boyfriend.

MS. N: I never felt like I was getting the affection I needed from him, and I was doing so much for him! It felt so unfair. Then I started to get very anxious just thinking about him. Not quite panic, though.

THERAPIST: What do you think made you anxious?

MS. N: It was confusing. I was so mad at him that I wanted to break up with him, but I wasn't sure. Then I was worrying that he was going to reject me if I got angry!

THERAPIST: Did you tell him how you were feeling?

MS. N: Not really because I was worried I would start yelling at him, and that would make things even worse.

The therapist's exploration indicated that, in addition to a patient's death, both her work and close relationships contributed to Ms. N's increasing anxiety and panic. In addition, the evaluation suggested that, dynamically, she had a pervasive sense of unfairness (at work and with her former boyfriend) and a conflict about her angry feelings, as with her boyfriend. For example, she feared that her anger would disrupt her relationship with her boyfriend, consistent with dynamic factors found in panic disorder (Busch et al., 2012). Further exploration (*again, using the guiding questions from Worksheet 3.4, pp. 80–81*) revealed that her early experiences with a temperamental father and anxious mother contributed to these fears.

THERAPIST: Can you describe your parents? What were they like?

MS. N: My dad is a little on the tense side. That's just his nature. He would come home from work, and he'd be upset, and he would yell and take it out on us. And I would say, "Why is he yelling at mommy?" My mom is very nervous: She panics. Not an actual panic attack, but she worries about everything.

THERAPIST: Can you describe your parents' attitudes and behavior toward you? Did you consider your early environment abusive or neglectful in any way?

MS. N: My father would slap me on occasion. I don't think that's abusive, though. He would hit me in the face if I was really bad. Nothing that left a mark or anything.

Identifying Situations, Emotions, and Thoughts

THERAPIST: How were anxiety and separations managed in the family?

MS. N: My mother was always terrified that something bad would happen to us if we were out late—especially if my father found out.

THERAPIST: How was anger managed in the family?

MS. N: My father had a terrible temper. Everyone was afraid of him.

THERAPIST: Did your parents fight? How much? About what?

MS. N: They wouldn't fight because my mother was very fearful of displeasing my father. He would get so mad at her.

THERAPIST: What were your siblings like? What were your experiences with your siblings?

MS. N: My younger sister is kind of a leader with me. She's very attractive and outgoing. My parents treated me as the youngest. And I felt I got the short end of the stick. It was very unfair.

THERAPIST: Were there other significant caregivers in your early life (e.g., grandparents, nanny)?

MS. N: My grandparents were nice, but I hardly ever saw them.

THERAPIST: What was the environment you grew up in like (cultural, religious, financial, etc.)?

MS. N: I'm from a Catholic background, middle class. I think I'm very prone to guilt from that. I felt guilty about how angry I was at my boyfriend.

THERAPIST: Did you experience any major losses or injuries growing up?

MS. N: Not that I recall.

THERAPIST: Did you have any experiences you would consider traumatic growing up?

MS. N: I guess I hadn't thought of it before but now I feel I wasn't treated very well because my father had such a bad temper and my mother was so nervous. Also, it wasn't very fair how they treated my sister as if she were the older one. But I don't know if that was trauma.

As they reviewed this worksheet and her history, Ms. N and the therapist were able to make clear connections between her temperamental and anxious family, her sense of unfairness, and her fears of her anger. In this context, Ms. N acknowledged a broader understanding of the origins of her panic rather than just recent stresses: "I guess I'm just an anxious person. I realize my family was nervous and scary. Our parents were on edge, so it's normal to be anxious and worrying. I'm learning through therapy why I've been that way. It does stem back to a very young age. At first, I thought, 'Oh, I panicked because I saw somebody die.' But now I understand it wasn't just that one incident. I think it's just a long process, a lot of feelings, and things you just keep inside of you. And then I was so frustrated and scared at work and with my boyfriend. I think the panic attacks were just all those things adding up and becoming too much!"

The chapters that follow demonstrate how developmental factors and current contexts, feelings, and thoughts are combined with an additional understanding of the patient's psychology in the form of a psychodynamic formulation. The formulation becomes a framework used for further intervention with specific problems.

QUESTIONS AND IDEAS TO THINK ABOUT

1. In addition to using PrFPP as a primary treatment intervention, these techniques can be used to address problems in current patients you have where you are using other treatment modalities, such as CBT or medication. If certain problems have persisted, consider evaluating the contexts, thoughts, and feelings surrounding these problems and developmental factors that may contribute. After trying this approach, can you describe what you and the patient learned from this exploration?

2. Consider the personal issues that you struggle with in your life (e.g., temper episodes, anxious periods), considering the contexts, feelings, and thoughts that exacerbate them. What factors in your own history may be contributory? Do you think awareness of these factors could help you to better manage them?

HANDOUT 3.1

Paying Attention to Circumstances, Thoughts, Feelings, and Reactions Associated with Problems

An important way to understand what contributes to your problems and how to fix them is learning to monitor your thoughts, feelings, behaviors, and circumstances that trigger their onset or worsening. Mostly, people are unaware or do not really attend to what they are experiencing at the start or exacerbation of their problems. Monitoring your thoughts, feelings, and stresses can help determine contributors to problems and work to diminish them. It also helps you find ways to step back and observe your problems rather than feel caught up in them. It may be useful to use a diary that your therapist will provide to write down what you experience when your problem worsens. This diary can help to practice your skills of self-observation and provide your therapist with information to develop strategies for addressing your problems.

From *Skills Training in Psychodynamic Psychotherapy*, by Fredric N. Busch. Copyright © 2026 The Guilford Press. Permission to photocopy this handout, or to download and print additional copies (*www.guilford.com/busch-forms*), is granted to purchasers of this book for personal use or use with clients; see copyright page for details.

WORKSHEET 3.1

Monitoring Circumstances, Thoughts, Feelings, and Reactions Surrounding Problems

Below is a diary to help monitor your problems and relevant triggers. Make a notation in your diary whenever you observe the onset or worsening of a problem. Keeping such a log of these experiences will aid you in developing the capacity to attend to the problems that are troubling you and begin to define the stressors, emotions, and thoughts that contribute to them (see examples inserted below).

Date	*Circumstances* Describe what was happening at that time.	*Thoughts*	*Feelings*	*Reactions* Describe how you reacted.

From *Skills Training in Psychodynamic Psychotherapy*, by Fredric N. Busch. Copyright © 2026 The Guilford Press. Permission to photocopy this worksheet, or to download and print additional copies (*www.guilford.com/busch-forms*), is granted to purchasers of this book for personal use or use with clients; see copyright page for details.

WORKSHEET 3.2

Assessing Triggers and Content of Panic Attacks

These questions will help you and your therapist gather information about the underlying causes that may trigger your panic attacks.

What kinds of feelings or experiences did you notice preceded your panic?

Can you give me the details of a specific trigger?

What thoughts and fears accompanied your panic?

Do you have a sense of other problems, tensions, or past experiences in your life that may contribute to these fears?

From *Skills Training in Psychodynamic Psychotherapy*, by Fredric N. Busch. Copyright © 2026 The Guilford Press. Permission to photocopy this worksheet, or to download and print additional copies (*www.guilford.com/busch-forms*), is granted to purchasers of this book for personal use or use with clients; see copyright page for details.

WORKSHEET 3.3

Exploring Not Acting on an Impulsive Behavior

The questions below will help you explore what it would feel like to not act on an impulsive behavior.

If you imagine not acting on the impulse to behave in this way, what do you think will happen or that you'll experience?

Are you certain that you'll have a negative reaction?

How do you feel when you've acted on the impulse?

(continued)

From *Skills Training in Psychodynamic Psychotherapy*, by Fredric N. Busch. Copyright © 2026 The Guilford Press. Permission to photocopy this worksheet, or to download and print additional copies (*www.guilford.com/busch-forms*), is granted to purchasers of this book for personal use or use with clients; see copyright page for details.

Exploring Not Acting on an Impulsive Behavior *(page 2 of 2)*

How would it feel to try holding off acting on the impulse as a test to see what will happen?

If you made this attempt to delay, what thoughts and feelings did you have when you held off acting on the impulse?

Are you willing to try it again?

WORKSHEET 3.4

Exploring Enacting an Inhibited Behavior

The questions below will help you explore what it would feel like to enact a behavior you have been inhibited from doing.

If you imagine enacting an inhibited behavior, what do you think will happen or that you'll experience?

Are you certain that you'll have a negative reaction?

How do you feel when you avoid enacting the behavior?

(continued)

From *Skills Training in Psychodynamic Psychotherapy*, by Fredric N. Busch. Copyright © 2026 The Guilford Press. Permission to photocopy this worksheet, or to download and print additional copies (www.guilford.com/busch-forms), is granted to purchasers of this book for personal use or use with clients; see copyright page for details.

Exploring Enacting an Inhibited Behavior (page 2 of 2)

How would it feel to try enacting the behavior as a test to see what will happen?

If you made this attempt to enact the behavior, what thoughts and feelings did you have afterward?

Are you willing to try it again?

WORKSHEET 3.5
Exploring Developmental History

These questions will help you and your therapist gather information to help you understand the sources of your problems in order to better address and manage them.

Can you describe your parents? What were they like?

Can you describe your parents' attitudes and behavior toward you? Did you consider your early environment abusive or neglectful in any way?

How were anxiety and separations managed in the family?

(continued)

From *Skills Training in Psychodynamic Psychotherapy*, by Fredric N. Busch. Copyright © 2026 The Guilford Press. Permission to photocopy this worksheet, or to download and print additional copies (*www.guilford.com/busch-forms*), is granted to purchasers of this book for personal use or use with clients; see copyright page for details.

Exploring Developmental History *(page 2 of 3)*

How was anger managed in the family?

Did your parents fight? How much? About what?

What were your siblings like? What were your experiences with your siblings?

Were there other significant caregivers in your early life (e.g., grandparents, nanny)?

(continued)

Exploring Developmental History *(page 3 of 3)*

What was the environment you grew up in like (cultural, religious, financial, etc.)?

Did you experience any major losses or injuries growing up?

Did you have any experiences you would consider traumatic growing up?

CHAPTER 4

Identifying and Addressing Self and Other Representations

As noted in Chapter 1, individuals have inner mental **representations and models of interactions between themselves and others**, predominantly deriving from significant developmental experiences and relationships (Bowlby, 1973; Jacobson, 1964), as well as temperamental factors. As noted, these models are part of the object relations theory of psychoanalysis. The nature of these models plays an important role in the emergence of symptoms and problems, as they affect the way people view themselves and what they anticipate from others. For example, if individuals see themselves as inadequate and others as judgmental, they will have a propensity to judge themselves poorly and expect or perceive criticism from others. Individuals who have self-representations of inadequacy and representations of others as being critical, rejecting, or attacking will tend to experience low self-esteem and social anxiety. Thus, identifying these **self and other representations** is important to understanding and addressing their contributions to problems.

Clinicians obtain information about self and other representations by listening for patterns of how patients describe themselves and others, as well as their anticipated and actual interpersonal interactions. To the extent that there is a rigidity and negativity in their representations, they are more likely to be related to problem areas. Descriptions of developmental experiences with significant attachment figures are considered particularly relevant for understanding the origins of self and other representations. Thus, it is important for patients to realize that they may be anticipating a high level of negative representations and interactions based on past developmental experiences rather than their current circumstances. In this chapter, numerous clinical examples are provided that describe such constellations and interventions designed to address them. The chapter concludes with a review of a developing psychodynamic formulation and interventions that can be derived from the increasing understanding of patients' problems and their triggers, their developmental history, and their self and other representations.

SELF AND OTHER REPRESENTATIONS: HOW YOU SEE AND WHAT YOU EXPECT FROM YOURSELF AND OTHERS

Therapists can use the questions on Worksheet 4.1: Self and Other Representations: How You See and What You Expect from Yourself and Others (pp. 104–106) to initially explore the patient's self and other representations. (All worksheets are available online at *www.guilford.com/busch-forms*.)

In the session, you might explain to your patient that responding to these questions will shed light on their problems by getting more specific about how they view themselves and what they expect from others. You can use the questions as a guide for your clinical interview, or you can give them the worksheet, saying, "In the next few days, before our next session, I'd like you to try completing this worksheet. It asks you to try describing the ways you predominantly see yourself and what you anticipate from others." Their responses can then be used as a basis for further exploration of their self and other representations.

The following case demonstrates the use of this worksheet with a patient who suffered severe recurrent depression and severe trauma in childhood.

CASE EXAMPLE: MR. O

Mr. O was a divorced 46-year-old White lawyer who presented for treatment with severe recurrent major depression and who entered PrFPP treatment along with a series of antidepressant trials. His depressive preoccupations focused on how he experienced himself as a failure and felt badly treated by the law firms he had worked for. Upon exploration of his history, Mr. O described his father, a successful entrepreneur, as a bully, who had high intellectual expectations and a harsh response about his son's inability to meet them. His father would castigate and humiliate him, calling him a "loser" and "nobody's genius" when he could not answer certain questions. He had difficulty tolerating the high regard in which his father was held by the community and family members for his business successes, knowing how his father behaved at home. As he was approaching adolescence, he became aware that his father was behaving increasingly erratically and retrospectively suspected that his father was using drugs. At age 12, Mr. O witnessed the sudden death of his father from a heart attack. His immediate response was complicated in that he felt relief in addition to guilt that he had somehow contributed to his father's death.

Upon entering therapy, Mr. O minimized the impact of his father's death on his current problems. However, evidence suggested that he had developed chronically low self-esteem since childhood and significant conflict about his aggressive and competitive wishes. This conflict emerged in a pattern in which his work successes were followed by guilt, anxiety, and the anticipation of a punitive response from superiors. At these times, he demonstrated self-destructive behavior, acting in ways that would provoke a negative response, such as getting into fights with senior partners about how to handle cases. These conflicts were so severe that he lost two different jobs, and he began to struggle with maintaining employment, despite his significant skill set. Ultimately, he had to take a job at a small firm rather than the well-known large firms at which he previously worked. This "demotion" led to a surge in depressive symptoms, with intense self-criticism and a view of himself as a failure, leading him to seek treatment.

Mr. O reported that, preceding his father's death and even more so after, his mother was unresponsive to his needs and was unempathic regarding the impact of the loss of his father. She probably suffered from an undiagnosed chronic depression. His older brother and sister were spared the worst of his father's tirades and were not at home when he died; neither of them suffered similar recurrent depressive episodes. Mr. O had divorced 5 years previously after chronic struggles with his wife, but he did have a fairly close relationship with his 16-year-old daughter. He had not dated for some time, believing that "women would not be interested in me." He gave the following responses to Worksheet 4.1 (pp. 104–106) on self and other representations:

Describe the ways you see yourself.

I see myself as having failed at everything, even though I was successful in my jobs at first.

In what ways do you feel negatively about yourself?

I've never really achieved anything. All I can do is this low-level job.

What intensifies or triggers negative views about yourself?

When I apply for a job at a large firm and get no response. Or if a friend doesn't get back to me when I've told him I need help finding a job.

Do you feel that you should be punished for something you thought or did?

Yes. When my father fell on the floor, for a while I didn't say anything. I was just stunned, but I didn't want him around. I still feel guilty about that, and I still feel relieved.

Do you find that you are always raising the bar?

No. I think I have a reasonable bar set, but others might say they're high expectations.

Describe how you think others see you.

I think others see me as a failure or maybe don't even care about me. This includes my very successful siblings. My daughter seems to care about me, but I'm not sure why.

What kinds of responses do you anticipate from others? What kinds of needs do you express toward them?

I pretty much expect others at this point to just dismiss me. So, I don't ask for much. And when I do, I don't get much back. Like help finding a job.

How often do you feel that your expectations are accurate?

I think that the lack of response I expect is pretty much what happens. People just don't want to have much to do with me. In fact, I hardly contact old friends because I feel they won't have interest now that I'm not at a well-known firm.

Do you idealize others? Has this led you to become disappointed in them? Do you compare yourself unfavorably to them?

I certainly compare myself unfavorably to others, but I don't idealize them. There were some people who were supportive of me early in my legal career whom I admire.

After reading Mr. O's responses to the worksheet, the therapist explored further how these self and other representations affected him and began to challenge them:

THERAPIST: You clearly view yourself quite negatively and anticipate that others will either be critical or disregard you. You seem to completely ignore successes.

MR. O: It's clear that others don't want to have anything to do with me. I contacted my friend Tom, letting him know I was at this small firm but wasn't happy there. He said he might have a connection to a larger, better-known firm. He's a partner at firm X and very successful and busy. We met together and discussed some options. We were supposed to meet again, but now he hasn't gotten back to me to follow up. Clearly, I'm his lowest priority.

THERAPIST: You sound hurt and angry about this.

MR. O: I guess I'm getting kind of used to it. Maybe he heard I got into conflicts that led to me getting fired from my last two firms. But I can't stand being pushed around like this. I feel like writing to him and saying, "If you're not serious about it, just forget it."

THERAPIST: It seems to me there's a good chance that would push him away. Maybe when you feel hurt and mad, you push others away and end up feeling more alone. Maybe you could just ask him when he might get back to you.

MR. O: Maybe. I try to watch out about getting angry and distancing others. But I'm also afraid to ask him.

THERAPIST: Why is that?

MR. O: I'm afraid I'll find out for sure he doesn't have any ideas for me.

THERAPIST: You've got yourself in a trap, as either way you end up feeling rejected. And you assume that he's disregarding you, like you felt with your mother, and that it's not possible that he's just busy and having trouble getting around to it.

MR. O: Yeah, I definitely don't think about it that way.

This exploration demonstrates how Mr. O's predominant self and other representations added to low self-esteem with feelings of failure and depression, as well as a persistent tendency to get into struggles with others. In this exchange, the therapist demonstrates how he is beginning to address these representations, indicating the degree to which the patient is excessively negative and linking them to his early life experiences.

Formulating Self and Other Representations

As part of the psychodynamic formulation for a given case, the therapist identifies a set of self and other representations for each patient, working with patients to recognize their views and expectations of themselves and others. This formulation also provides a framework for the therapist to address these representations by identifying where they derive from and pointing out inaccuracies and contradictions. For example, based on the information obtained above the therapist suggested the following self and other representations for Mr. O's psychodynamic formulation:

- Self as a failure, bad; others as judgmental, humiliating
- Self as unlovable; others as neglectful, uncaring
- Self as damaging to others in being assertive, competitive; others as punitive

In the formulation, self and other representations are typically paired, as a specific self-representation tends to match with a particular representation of others. The third representation for Mr. O refers to his guilt and expectation of punishment in being assertive or competitive. Ultimately, this conflict was found to be related to guilty feelings regarding the relief he felt in "defeating" his father, by somehow contributing to his death. Subsequent cases in this chapter further describe approaches targeting these self and other representations. The therapist looks for these self and other representations to shift in a positive direction as treatment proceeds.

CASE EXAMPLE: MS. P'S FEARS OF REJECTION AND PRESSURE TO CARE FOR OTHERS

Ms. P was a 52-year-old White married woman and mother of four, with her own small public relations firm, who developed depressive symptoms after her last child went to college. She felt frustrated with the level of success of her company and "bored" with her husband and friends. At this point, she developed a flirtation with a younger man, Eric, who had a job as a salesman in one of the companies she worked for. She became excited and sexually attracted to him, intensified by his inviting her to do "fun" activities that her husband was not interested in, such as surfing and sailing. However, she was unwilling to have sex with Eric, out of concern about her marriage, which was quite frustrating to him. Indeed, Eric would pull back from the relationship after she rebuffed his advances, although he did not say why he was withdrawing.

Rather than consider the possibility that Eric was distancing himself from her because of the boundaries she set on their relationship, she was convinced that he had met a new girlfriend and was no longer interested in her, creating severe anxiety and a down mood. However, shortly after Eric pulled back from the relationship, he resumed pursuing her. Despite his reengagement, she was left in an anxious state as to whether he would abruptly pull back again, this time for good.

At the same time, Ms. P felt pressure to take care of others at the expense of her own needs. A prime example involved her niece Claire, who had significant financial problems and suffered from anxiety and depression. Ms. P felt guilty about her brother's poor parenting of his niece, as he struggled with finding work, was divorced from Claire's mother, and had little contact with Claire. Ms. P gave her both financial support and a job, hiring Claire to work for her company. However, Claire would often miss work, citing multiple somatic complaints. This would require Ms. P to take over her tasks until her return, creating significant stress and adding to her anxiety and depression.

Her therapist raised the question of why Ms. P persisted in this caretaking behavior. In exploring these pressures, it emerged that she felt guilty if she did not support others, worrying that if she did not care for them, they could fall apart. The patient also feared losing attachment to the others if they became angry about her withdrawing support. In this view, Ms. P believed that others were only focused on getting their own needs met and did not care about her.

Given Ms. P's perceptions of self and others, along with her proneness to anxiety and depression, the therapist developed the following formulation of her self and other representations:

- Self as on the verge of rejection; others as not dependable, rejecting
- Self as responsible for others' well-being; others as fragile
- Self as needing to care for others to maintain attachment; others as self-focused

Identifying Self and Other Representations and Their Relationship to Problems

A key step in the therapeutic process of PrFPP is linking the self and other representations that are identified to the specific problems patients are struggling with. One important aspect of this approach is helping patients recognize these contributors to their problems, giving them potential control over these issues by understanding the factors contributing to them. A second component is giving patients a framework for targeting problems, providing relief by addressing negative self and other representations. What follows here are clinical examples illustrating this work in action. The first examples show the therapist making the links of self and other representations to problems; the subsequent examples show the therapist addressing negative self and other representations.

Linking Self and Other Representations to Problems

CASE EXAMPLE 1: MR. O

In addressing the problems of Mr. O, the therapist linked his self and other representations to his feelings of painful depression, humiliation, and social isolation in several ways. These included his self-view of being a failure and his anticipation that others would reject, criticize, or humiliate him. In addition, the threat he anticipated from others by competing and asserting himself led him to unconsciously undermine his efforts by precipitating interpersonal conflicts. This tendency triggered recurrent job losses that further reduced his self-esteem and increased his sense of helplessness, outrage, and victimization.

CASE EXAMPLE 2: MR. F

For Mr. F, who was driven to work excessively (see Chapter 2), his primary representations involved a view of himself as inadequate and a loser and others as demanding, judgmental, and critical. He attempted to compensate for these representations by pressuring himself to achieve, pushing himself to attain an elusive goal of satisfying his father's standards. This led to persistent anxiety in his efforts to meet an undefinable goal of success to gain a sense of value. This pressure then added to the problems involving disruptions with his family through his being overly focused on work.

CASE EXAMPLE 3: MR. A

As described previously (Chapter 1), Mr. A suffered predominantly from anxiety and panic attacks. Contributors to his panic episodes included fear of rejection and aloneness on the one hand and alternately feeling trapped by others' needs on the other. His self and other representations were identified by his therapist as the following:

- Self as socially inadequate, alone; others as rejecting
- Self as distressed by intrusion, control; others as controlling, intrusive

The latter set of representations around feeling trapped occurred during the following panic episode and were addressed by the therapist:

MR. A: I was playing tennis with my friend. He gets into political rants, and although I agree with him, I just get tired hearing them all the time. I felt like I wanted to get out of there, but I couldn't say anything. All of a sudden, I had an intense feeling of panic. I got down on the ground and gripped at my chest because it hurt. Kind of scared my friend, but I explained I had panic like this before.

THERAPIST: That sounds like a terrible episode. What do you mean you couldn't say anything?

MR. A: Well, it would be harsh if you were to tell a friend, "I just need to get away from you." That would be really hurtful.

THERAPIST: It sounds like in this case you felt trapped. You couldn't really say anything to get out of the situation but felt frightened and controlled being in it. But I'm wondering why you think you couldn't say anything, even if it were to say you're not feeling well and need a break, or even to make a joke about him being so focused on political rants.

MR. A: That's interesting because I have made joking comments to him at times about it, but this time I felt stuck.

THERAPIST: I wonder if you felt so worried about hurting him that it overrode your ability to think about it, and it sent you into a panic.

MR. A: That makes sense.

This pattern also indicates a conflict about aggression associated with assertiveness that is discussed further in Chapter 5. Additionally, it suggests another set of self and other representations: that of himself as potentially damaging to others and others as vulnerable.

CASE EXAMPLE 4: MS. P

Ms. P's depressive symptoms were notably related to her expectation of rejection by Eric and the pressure she felt to care for others. Both factors interfered with efforts to address the problems with her niece, to whom she yielded her own needs, and look for other sources of enjoyment.

THERAPIST: It really puts you in a difficult position to have your niece working for you.

MS. P: I know, but I'm not sure what to do because she'll fall apart otherwise.

THERAPIST: What do you think would happen to her?

MS. P: I hadn't really thought about that. She's not going to starve. I guess just get more anxious? Or maybe get mad and not talk to me? But I'm not sure. Maybe if I didn't make it easy for her, she'd actually do more work.

THERAPIST: It sounds like your worries are related to how you felt growing up, that your mother disengaged from parenting, and you felt your siblings would fall apart if you didn't take care of things. And you keep applying these same expectations to others.

MS. P: I guess it's possible. I hadn't looked at it that way.

The therapist's interpretation derived from exploring Ms. P's childhood, as described in the next section.

Linking Self and Other Representations to Developmental History

Linking self and other representations to developmental events performs several important functions. The first is to gain an understanding of the origins of these self and other representations. The second is to identify how they continue to influence patients in a significant, often unconscious, way. A third is to begin to differentiate current experiences and representations from those that emerged in the past. And the fourth is to use revisions of old representations to address problems.

CASE EXAMPLE: MS. P

In examining how Ms. P's development contributed to her representations, she described a neglectful early environment in which her father was absent frequently on business and her mother was self-focused, concentrating on social activities. Ms. P reported spending an inordinate amount of time at home alone, caring for her younger brother and sister. She described how she would sometimes need to scrounge for food in the house, even though her parents were in reasonable financial condition, as they neglected to go shopping. When she was age 10, her parents separated and divorced, and her father's new partner refused to allow visits with his children. Her mother had a series of boyfriends, many of whom the patient met.

As she grew up, she imagined her parents "having fun" while she did what she could to take care of her siblings and herself. She did gain a significant degree of interest from boys, which was a source of excitement and self-esteem for her, but often could not arrange to go out with them. Despite her caretaking efforts, her sister developed severe substance abuse problems, and her brother struggled in school, later going from job to job, with persistent financial difficulties. She attempted to help him with financial support and by hiring her niece. Ms. P's fears of abandonment and pressure to take care of others emerged from the neglect and disregard she felt from her parents, and the responsibility she felt to care for her younger siblings. The therapist was able to link these experiences with Ms. P's belief that Eric was on the verge of getting a "fun" girlfriend, with her being excluded and rejected. Additionally, she agreed with a connection the therapist suggested between pressures with her siblings growing up and her view that others needed her to take care of them to be okay.

Therapists can use the following guiding questions to identify how much patients are aware of the relationship between their early experiences and their self and other representations (see Worksheet 4.2: Linking Self and Other Representations to Early Experiences: Consider How You Felt with Your Caregivers When You Were Growing Up, pp. 107–108). As described earlier, in the session you might explain to your patient how you are trying to help them find links between their self and other representations and their past experiences. You can introduce the questions that follow, and then give them the worksheet, suggesting they fill it out in the days before your next session. These questions provide a way for patients to think about these links. The therapist should consider following up after sessions in which these links are identified to assess what information patients have gained.

For instance, Ms. P's responses to Worksheet 4.2 demonstrate a growing understanding of the origin and relevance of her self and other representations.

How did your parents (or other caregivers) see you, and what was your relationship with them?

I felt like more of a burden to them than anything else. They were really interested in their own activities. I'm not sure they wanted to have kids.

What did you expect from them? Where did they meet these expectations, and where did they fall short?

At first, I thought that this was just normal. But then when I met other kids' parents, I realized that something was really wrong. Sometimes I even had to scrounge around for food. I would have hoped for just some basic interest in us.

Do you see any connection or overlap between how you see yourself now and how your parents viewed you?

I never realized it before, but in therapy, the connection has become clearer. I assume that others aren't going to be interested in me unless I make a special effort to get them interested.

Do you see any connection or overlap between how you view others now and how you viewed your parents?

Again, I'm still working on this, but it seems like I just kind of expect others to reject me. And I feel like I have to take care of others to keep them around.

To the extent that you view yourself negatively, how might it be connected to early life experiences?

I don't really view myself negatively in general. But I guess I do to some extent if I just think other people are going to reject me.

Viewing Oneself as a Failure

Linking one's negative self-views, including feelings of failure, to developmental experiences is important for patients' being able to recognize and address these often persistent problems. In Mr. M's case, discussed in Chapter 3, the therapist and he had made a clear connection of the perception of himself as "bad" to his parents' view of him, with an expectation that he would be rejected or punished by others. Similarly, Mr. O's internalized view of himself as a "failure" or "loser" were essentially equivalent to the attitude and attacks he experienced from his father. Indeed, he appeared to accept these perceptions as valid despite his intense criticisms of his father (please see dissociated self and other representations below).

In these cases, significant compensatory efforts at success or, in Mr. M's case, to be "good" represented attempts to make up for these negative self-views. In Jacobson's (1971) theory, developed for depressive disorders, such compensatory efforts can create unreachable standards that invariably lead to a sense of falling short. Mr. F (the "workaholic" described in Chapter 2), for example, viewed himself as a loser despite the financial success he achieved by accepting all new clients, a tactic that created enormous self-pressure. Mr. F demonstrated the following self and other representations in relation to these efforts: self as a failure in achieving goals; others as demanding and impossible to please. In these instances, the sense of being a failure becomes part of the individual's representations in a way that is unmodifiable by their actual accomplishments. In addressing this form of self and other representations, the therapist communicates that an impossible standard has been established and helps the patient identify and take satisfaction or pride in what has been accomplished. Recognizing excessive self-expectations helps patients understand why they continue to feel like a failure despite their achievements. This challenge to negative representations may be particularly difficult in patients with a history of significant past trauma, such as Mr. O, who harshly dismissed the value of his past work accomplishments and his positive relationship with his daughter.

Feeling Trapped

In relation to feeling trapped, Mr. A recalled being harangued by his father, who focused on his professional struggles. His father demonstrated a lack of concern about the patient's life, including Mr. A's own interests. He recalled being frustrated by these "lectures" but unable to excuse himself, as his father would lose his temper if interrupted.

Although his mother attended to his father's speeches, she put pressure on Mr. A to respond to her own needs for attention, often complaining about his father, which made him very uncomfortable. Mr. A agreed that his anxiety and anger at feeling "trapped" by his friend's expectations were linked to these experiences with his parents. He would misread current situations as being trapped by others' needs with a fear of expressing his wishes to get distance.

Challenging Negative Self and Other Representations

As self and other representations and their link to problems and developmental factors are identified, the therapist focuses on challenging these negative representations and expectations and replacing them, where indicated, with more positive ones. Instead of this being a generalized effort, the therapist works on addressing the precise nature of negative views of self and others and specific evidence to counter them. Examples are given for the cases of Mr. O, Mr. M, and Mr. P. In challenging Mr. O's view of himself as a failure, it was evident that, while this sense of himself was global, his struggles related more to problems with his career than with his daughter. It became clear that Mr. O equated self-esteem with expectations of extraordinary and persistent work achievements. As he had not sustained this, he was a failure, ignoring his career successes. One approach to this self-view was to call attention to his achievements at the prestigious firms at which he worked before his relationships soured. The therapist also noted that he continued to earn the money he needed at the smaller firm, even though he felt devalued being there. In addition, therapist and patient explored how he often misread others as demeaning him when they were simply communicating to him tasks he needed to take care of, triggering the intense anger that led to disruptions with colleagues.

Information regarding his father's attitudes and behavior were considered relevant to Mr. O's problems, and the therapist linked these experiences with his highly negative and rigid representations. These included his father's disparaging of his intelligence and focus on school and career success. Indeed, his father had a meteoric rise in his profession but was reprimanded repeatedly for bullying and demeaning behavior toward his employees and colleagues. He referred to Mr. O as a failure and loser, and Mr. O believed that he could never meet his father's standards of what it meant to be successful in his work. His father saw no role in emotional care and support of his children, though he did emphasize financial success. The therapist pointed out that Mr. O had reflexively adopted his father's view in assessing his own value, even though he deeply disagreed and was furious with the way he was treated by his father. His mother's neglect and lack of interest in who he was as a person further added to his anger and feelings of failure.

As he continued to make efforts to deepen his relationship with his daughter, the therapist noted how different his behavior was from his father's as a parent and his daughter's close relationship with him. The therapist raised the point that he had a valuable role as a father that his own father never achieved. Although the patient maintained that he still felt worthless and that he was not that important to his daughter, a shift occurred when his daughter, who lived in another city, asked him to move nearby:

MR. O: My daughter asked me to move near her.

THERAPIST: How do you explain that, given the negative view you have of yourself?

MR. O: I don't get it, especially when I asked her and she said, "You're family." I mean to me being family isn't such a great thing.

THERAPIST: It seems obvious that she would like to have you living nearby because you're important to her.

MR. O: Okay, but it's very hard for me to believe that, especially given my failures in life.

THERAPIST: You seem to have adopted your father's view that a person's value depends entirely on career success, and yet your daughter doesn't see things in that way. She doesn't believe that a person's value stems entirely from career achievement.

MR. O: I find it hard to believe. But with my father, career achievement was the thing, though in the end he didn't really do so well at taking care of himself. So, his big career was cut short.

For Mr. M, his feeling of being a "bad" person was a central contributor to his anxiety and depression and needed to be targeted in the therapy. He recognized, with his therapist's help, that his parents saw his boyish rebellion as "bad," but somehow they had generalized this view of him in a way that felt hurtful and rejecting. The therapist and he challenged this notion of being bad by emphasizing his significant success with his business, his generosity to his employees and his ex-wife, and his efforts to help his children. Mr. M would become tearful when considering these factors, stating, "I guess I'm really not bad."

In the case of Ms. P, the therapist suggested that, in most instances, she did not have to take care of others for them to be okay and created a difficult burden for herself by doing so. In fact, the therapist averred, it may be better for others to learn to manage themselves: Taking care of her niece may inadvertently be rewarding her dependent behavior. In considering the developmental origin of these representations, the therapist suggested that Ms. P's pressure to support others stemmed from the necessity she felt to care for her younger siblings when her parents were neglectful. While indeed those efforts may have felt or been essential at that time, her niece was an adult and not in the same dependent position. Ms. P began to step back from taking care of her niece, which did not lead to her niece's collapse or withdrawal from her. Indeed, while expressing annoyance at Ms. P for being "withholding," her niece began to make greater efforts in her work and self-care.

In addressing her expectations of rejection by others, the therapist suggested Ms. P's likely role in Eric's withdrawal. Ms. P had trouble considering the possibility that

Eric's distancing himself was in part secondary to limits she set on the relationship. In addition, the therapist and she, using the approach of mentalization (see Chapters 1 and 6), discussed how Eric, who was in his early 40s, had never had a long-term relationship with a woman and appeared to have trouble with commitment. In fact, he told her that, in the year prior to meeting her, he had had two or three different girlfriends with the relationships lasting only a month or two.

In the case of Mr. A, the therapist explored the pressure he felt to respond to the needs of others, which included a belief that he was socially inadequate. Stories he told of his interactions with others suggested that he was quite sought after and effective socially, and others viewed him as thoughtful and amusing. The therapist also explored the danger that Mr. A felt if he raised his own needs or frustrations with others. They were able to link this fear to his early experiences with his father, noting how he assumed that others would be as self-focused or angry as his father was if he brought up his concerns. Successes in raising his own wishes, including with his husband and a friend, helped diminish the threat and anxiety he experienced.

Developing Specific Thoughts to Counter Self and Other Representations

Because self and other representations operate at a reflexive or unconscious level, they can be difficult to change consistently and tend to snap back into operation outside of the patient's awareness. For example, Ms. P's constant need to take responsibility for others, particularly her niece and younger brother and sister, would ease temporarily after discussing it, followed by the return of her usual pressures and behavior. Addressing intrapsychic conflicts and defenses (see Chapter 5) that contribute to the persistence of these representations is one key approach. But it can also be of value to work with the patient to develop an ongoing alertness to the presence of these self and other representations (perhaps using the circumstances/thoughts/feelings diary described in Chapter 3) and a list of thoughts to counter them. These specific counterthoughts and feelings are intended to address precise elements of the negative self and other representations. These interventions target aspects of the psychodynamic formulation for the patient's problems (see below). Below are some examples of this approach in the cases discussed in this chapter.

In challenging Mr. O's view of himself as a failure rejected by others, the therapist and he discussed the following way of thinking about it: "I know that I focus on achievement professionally because of my father's view, but it does count for something that I have such a positive relationship with my daughter. In fact, things are going so well that she asked me to move to the city she lives."

For Mr. M, the therapist worked to address the persistent notion of his being bad. The therapist and Mr. M identified the following reminder for him: "I feel that I'm bad, but actually I've had significant success in my business. In fact, I'm very generous to my employees and ex-wife, and have made important efforts to be closer to my kids."

For Ms. P, the therapist and she addressed her recurrent tendency to care for others with the following statement: "I don't have to take care of others for them to be okay. In fact, my niece is doing better since I've stepped back in my support for her." In the case of Eric, the therapist and she identified: "I know I tend to believe that I'm being rejected by others and that Eric would suddenly lose interest in me, but I recognize that he must be frustrated by the limits I've set on our relationship."

Dissociated Self and Other Representations

When self and other representations are dissociated (Busch, 2022, 2024), patients have polarized representations that can be contradictory, and yet these contradictions are not registered consciously. These dissociative patterns are quite common, particularly in relation to traumatic backgrounds (Busch, 2024). For instance, Mr. O was enraged at his father for his judgmental and humiliating behavior toward him and yet fully accepted his father's view of him as a failure. Once these representations are identified, the therapist can point out the contradiction between these modes. This identification will enable a process in which evidence can be brought forth to challenge these dissociated representations. In the case of Mr. O, the therapist noted how his acceptance of his father's view of him as a failure did not make sense in light of the intensely negative view he had of his father's values and attitudes.

Dissociated representations also add to difficulties managing anger at others, as in the case of Mr. O. A common developmental precursor of these dissociated states involves an intense desire to connect with abusive attachment figures, including controlling, critical, and/or neglectful/rejecting caregivers. Individuals experiencing such childhood maltreatment feel pressure to yield to parents' expectations to avoid attack or abandonment, alternating with conscious or unconscious rage at them. Such pressures can trigger development of a "false self" (Winnicott, 1965), submitting to others' expectations, alongside a self that rebels against these demands, while unaware of these shifts. These dissociated representations frequently lead patients to not recognize the adverse impact of their angry behavior (Busch, 2024). Mr. O, for example, would accept tasks he would see as devaluing, such as work paralegals could manage, but then feel enraged he was being asked to do work that was below his skill level.

MR. O: I'm struggling with this urge to blow up at the senior partner for giving me these low-level tasks, but I know that's going to get me into trouble. I shouldn't have accepted them in the first place.

THERAPIST: Did you have a choice?

MR. O: It depends on how you see it. He asked me if I would mind taking care of these things, as the paralegal was out sick. It's a small firm.

THERAPIST: Why did you agree to do it?

MR. O: Because I'm trying to be the "good boy" and not get in trouble. But now I'm recognizing this pattern where my rage gets me into trouble.

THERAPIST: That makes sense to look out for your anger and better understand it. You told me your pattern with the partners at the prior firms was to just accept how they handled cases and then, after your disagreements built up, get into a fight. It seems like you feel you have to submit to the authority, like with your father, but then you get increasingly enraged about doing that.

MR. O: I am becoming more aware of that problem. Thinking about it helped me settle down. I literally can't afford another temper outburst.

BUILDING A FORMULATION

At this point in the treatment, the therapist has identified a problem list, relevant developmental factors, a set of self and other representations, and a set of interventions. For purposes of PrFPP, the therapist can consider writing a beginning formulation that includes these elements. This will help the therapist track efforts to address problems using the formulation as a framework. There is also the option to share this with the patient or have the patient contribute to the formulation. Some examples taken from cases discussed in this chapter are as follows:

Problem List, Formulation, and Interventions for Mr. O

Problem list

1. Recurrent depression
2. Self-esteem sensitivity
3. Anger leading to disruptions at work
4. Fears of assertiveness

Self and other representations

Self as a failure; others as rejecting, judgmental
Self as unlovable; others as neglectful
Self as damaging; others as vulnerable

Developmental history

Father was self-focused, impulsive, and highly critical, with impossible standard for success. Mother was submissive to father and neglectful of the patient's emotional needs.

Interventions

Link his depression to feelings of failure, anger that become self-directed, and a lack of responsiveness of others (overall dynamics).

Connect patient's feelings of failure to father's harsh judgment and criticism (developmental link).

Link his sense of his unlovability and others' unresponsiveness to mother's neglect (developmental link).

Address how the patient disparages father's behavior and yet accepts father's criticism and view of him as a failure (developmental link/self and other representations).

Address patient's guilt about having damaged father (developmental link).

Address patient's fear of damaging others if he raised his concerns (self and other representations).

Challenge patient's overly negative self-view in light of his past work success and role as a parent (self and other representation).

Problem List, Formulation, and Interventions for Ms. P

Problem list

1. Depressive symptoms
2. Anxious symptoms
3. Fears of rejection
4. Pressure to respond to others' needs
5. Tensions in relationship with husband

Developmental history

Both parents were abandoning and neglectful of patient's needs, leading her to anticipate rejection. Pressure to take care of her younger siblings represented an attempt to please mother, keep siblings safe.

Self and other representations

Self as on the verge of rejection; others as not dependable, rejecting

Self as responsible for others' well-being; others as fragile

Self as needing to care for others to maintain attachment; others as self-focused

Interventions

Link expectations of rejection, need to yield her own needs to others to depressive and anxious symptoms (overall formulation).

Link patient's expectation of rejection to parents' neglect (developmental link).

Link need to care for others to pressure to care for younger siblings when growing up (developmental link).

Address patient's expectation of Eric rejecting her, not considering her limit setting with him (self and other representations).

Address patient's pressure to respond to others, yielding to their needs (self and other representations).

Address patient's acceptance of husband's lack of engagement (self and other representations).

Problem List, Formulation, and Interventions for Mr. A

Problem list

1. Panic attacks
2. Social anxiety
3. Anxiety when feeling pressured by others' demands
4. Tensions with husband, others around control, intrusiveness

Developmental history

Father was self-focused, lecturing about work, temperamental. Mother was anxious, demanding of patient's support.

Self and other representations

Self as socially inadequate; others as rejecting

Self as distressed by intrusion, control; others as controlling, intrusive

Interventions

Panic attacks as related to fear of isolation, as well as fears of being burdened by others' needs (overall formulation).

Link fears of being alone, trapped by father's self-focus, mother's emotional demands (developmental link).

Address fears of inadequacy socially when socially quite capable (self and other representations).

Link problems with husband to patient's fear of intrusiveness, control (self and other representations).

Address how ambivalence with husband intensified with separation, intrusion (address self and other representation).

A next step in the development of a psychodynamic formulation is identification and addressing of intrapsychic conflicts and defenses and how they further contribute to problems. These are described in the next chapter.

> **QUESTIONS AND IDEAS TO THINK ABOUT**
>
> 1. With one of your current patients, try identifying their predominant negative self and other representations. What interventions do you think would be able to address these?
> 2. With the same patient, try to identify where the representations derived from, particularly considering the patient's early experiences. How might you communicate such links in a useful way to the patient?

WORKSHEET 4.1

Self and Other Representations: How You See and What You Expect from Yourself and Others

These questions will help you and your therapist get more specific details about how you view and what you expect from yourself and others. This will help you and your therapist identify and address how your perceptions of yourself and others contribute to your problems.

How do you describe the ways you see yourself?

In what ways do you feel negatively about yourself?

What intensifies or triggers negative views about yourself?

(continued)

From *Skills Training in Psychodynamic Psychotherapy*, by Fredric N. Busch. Copyright © 2026 The Guilford Press. Permission to photocopy this worksheet, or to download and print additional copies (www.guilford.com/busch-forms), is granted to purchasers of this book for personal use or use with clients; see copyright page for details.

Self and Other Representations (page 2 of 3)

Do you feel that you should be punished for something you thought or did?

Do you find that you are always raising the bar?

Describe how you think others see you.

What kinds of needs do you express toward others? What kinds of responses do you anticipate from them?

(continued)

Self and Other Representations *(page 3 of 3)*

How often do you feel that your expectations are accurate?

Do you idealize others? Has this led you to become disappointed in them? Do you compare yourself unfavorably to them?

WORKSHEET 4.2

Linking Self and Other Representations to Early Experiences: Consider How You Felt with Your Caregivers When You Were Growing Up

These questions will help you and your therapist gather information in an effort to find links between your views and expectations of yourself and others and your past experiences. These links will help identify where negative perceptions of yourself and others derive from and how you and your therapist can address them.

How did your parents (or other caregivers) see you, and what was your relationship with them?

What did you expect from them? Where did they meet these expectations, and where did they fall short?

Do you see any connection or overlap between how you see yourself now and how your parents viewed you?

(continued)

From *Skills Training in Psychodynamic Psychotherapy*, by Fredric N. Busch. Copyright © 2026 The Guilford Press. Permission to photocopy this worksheet, or to download and print additional copies (www.guilford.com/busch-forms), is granted to purchasers of this book for personal use or use with clients; see copyright page for details.

Linking Self and Other Representations
to Early Experiences *(page 2 of 2)*

Do you see any connection or overlap between how you view others now and how you viewed your parents?

To the extent that you view yourself negatively, how might it be connected to early life experiences?

CHAPTER 5

Addressing Intrapsychic Conflicts and Defenses

Intrapsychic conflicts (defined in Chapter 1) involve wishes or impulses that are often unconscious and internalized prohibitions about them that lead them to feel unacceptable. These conflicts typically trigger anxiety and/or guilt due to fears of acting on these fantasies (Freud, 1926). Two wishes can also create conflict if they are experienced as contradictory, such as wanting to help and hurt someone. Intrapsychic conflict is common but can reach a level of severity that causes significant distress and contributes to an array of problems.

A key part of PrFPP is the identification of intrapsychic conflicts that patients struggle with and their link to specific problems. Once patients are aware of these conflicts, the therapist works to help better manage and tolerate them, to reduce associated symptoms and behavioral difficulties. Certain core wishes are common sources of conflict and problems, including fantasies or urges to harm others, wishes to be taken care of by others, and sexual desires. Conflicts about aggressive wishes, including those of hurting, controlling, or outdoing others, can lead to fears of damaging people that are important to the patient, potentially disrupting relationships or triggering retaliation. Thus, these wishes can cause anxiety or panic, particularly if the patient feels dependent on these individuals. This dynamic is commonly found in anxiety disorders, panic, and Cluster C personality disorders (Busch et al., 2012), although it can play a role in a wide array of problems. Such wishes can also cause guilt about harming others who are also loved. Conflicts about potentially damaging others can also lead to anger being directed toward the self in the form of self-attacks or self-punishment, a common dynamic in depressive symptoms. As is discussed in a later section of this chapter on defenses, conflicted anger can also be denied and viewed as coming from others (referred to as projection), who are

109

then inaccurately perceived as being attacking or rejecting, triggering anxiety, depression, and interpersonal problems.

Wishes to be close to or taken care of by others can create fears of rejection or intrusion, particularly if the individual has developmental experiences of abuse or neglect. Dependent wishes can be equated with weakness, which can lead to fears of exploitation or harm. This may lead to avoidance of intimate relationships or protective defenses such as denial of needing others. Sexual fantasies can cause guilt and anxiety if they are experienced as unacceptable or if there are urges to inappropriately act on them. Sexual wishes may also be linked to conflicted aggressive or intimate wishes, adding to conflict about the associated sexual fantasies. There are many forms of conflict in addition to those presented here: The therapist works to identify and address the conflicts related to the individual patient's problems.

Approaches to conflicts include identifying the specific nature of patients' wishes and their conflicts about them, as well as the dangers that patients anticipate. Next, therapists and patients work to identify the origins of these conflicts, particularly in the patient's developmental history, to better understand them. These steps become part of an effort to help patients tolerate their feelings and fantasies and work to build alternate ways of viewing them. An additional step includes finding ways to better manage these feelings and fantasies, both internally and in relationship to others.

IDENTIFYING INTRAPSYCHIC CONFLICTS

Although clinicians typically look for the emergence of these conflicts over the course of treatment, certain probes can give preliminary information about patients' propensity to these conflicts, as described in Worksheet 5.1: Conflicts about Feelings and Fantasies (pp. 128–129; all worksheets are available at *www.guilford.com/busch-forms*). In the session, you might explain to your patient that it will shed light on their problems to get more specific about feelings or wishes they have that cause them discomfort or feel threatening. You can use the questions presented as a guide for your clinical interview, or you can give them the worksheet, saying, "In the next few days, before our next session, I'd like you to try completing this worksheet. It asks you to try describing feelings and wishes that you have that cause you to feel anxious or guilty." Their responses can then be used as a basis for further exploration of their internal conflicts.

In the following section are sample answers that patients gave to these questions that indicate conflicts about these feelings and wishes.

Are you aware of any problems you have with angry feelings or expressing your anger?

I don't like expressing any anger because I don't like confrontation. I don't like fighting with people because I get worried that it will cause them to leave me. I usually just try to appease them.

I just don't think anger does you any good. I try to ignore those feelings when I have them.

When I get angry or vengeful I feel terribly guilty and end up getting angry at myself.

If I described my angry fantasies, you would find out what a terrible person I am.

I don't think there was any way I could get angry at my mother growing up. She had a furious temper, and she would lash back. She was scary and would sometimes hit us if we told her how we felt.

I wouldn't express anger at my mom because then she wouldn't talk to us for days. I get scared of the same thing happening now.

Sometimes I get so mad I get frightened that I'm going to act on these feelings.

I'm Catholic, and I believe that whatever revenge you seek you're going to end up getting punished for it.

Do you have fears about depending on other people?

I would like to depend on people, but I know you can't really trust them.

If you allow yourself to depend on other people, they'll take advantage of you.

I try depending on other people, but they always end up disappointing me.

To me, depending on others is a weakness. I feel I have to take care of myself.

Do you have fears about other people depending on you?

I feel pressured to take care of other people. If I don't do it, I feel guilty.

If I don't take care of other people, they'll fall apart.

Do you have fears about separating from others?

I know I have problems with my boyfriend, but if I break up with him, I'll feel completely alone.

I'm worried about trying to move away from home. I know I need to be more independent, but I really like my mom taking care of me.

Do you struggle with mixed feelings about others?

I want distance from my wife, but then when she goes away, I really miss her.

My sons seek out help from me, and part of me is like "Shouldn't you guys be on your own now?" But then I feel guilty. Shouldn't I want to take care of them? But then I feel pressured by them.

Are there any difficulties you have with your sexual feelings and fantasies?

My sexual fantasies sometimes involve my controlling and hurting other people. I feel guilty having them, and I wouldn't tell anyone about them. Of course, I would never act on them.

Sometimes I have sexual fantasies about men, and I feel I shouldn't be having those fantasies. Even though I don't feel negatively about gay people, somehow I still think it means I'm weak.

I have some fantasies where I submit sexually to a muscular man, but isn't it wrong to have these fantasies? I wouldn't want this to happen in real life.

Interventions for Areas of Conflict

A range of interventions is available for therapists to use to address intrapsychic conflict, including identifying them (interpretation) and helping patients better understand and tolerate their wishes and feelings. Below are some general comments therapists might make to relieve patients' conflicts about their fantasies:

It's normal for people to have such fantasies and feelings. It's how you act or don't act on them that's important.

The feelings and fantasies you have are quite understandable given what you experienced in your life.

Many people who have been victims of bullying have fantasies of bullying others, given what they experienced, but you can think about how you want to manage these fantasies.

For people who feel inhibited when they get angry, either because they feel guilty or worry that their anger will damage their relationships, it gets fraught trying to find effective ways to express it.

Despite your fears, anger can also have a positive value, by helping you address when you're being hurt or mistreated. However, it takes some work to sort out how to best modulate your anger and express it in an effective fashion.

CASE EXAMPLES OF IDENTIFYING AND ADDRESSING INTRAPSYCHIC CONFLICTS

The following case examples describe how therapists work to identify these conflicts and help patients feel more tolerant and better able to manage them. Developmental interpretations can also be helpful in this effort. Examples of conflicts about anger, separation/dependency, and sexuality are provided, including ways in which conflicts about these wishes and feelings interact.

Conflicts about Anger

Angry feelings and fantasies can be a significant area of conflict. Such conflicts can lead to fears of assertiveness, which can be inadvertently linked to anger, creating difficulties negotiating needs with others. Developmentally, conflicts over anger may be associated with identification with and fear of a caregiver with poorly managed anger.

CASE EXAMPLE: MR. Q'S CONFLICTED ANGER ABOUT BEING "MONITORED"

Mr. Q, a 49-year-old White married businessman, suffered from panic disorder and generalized anxiety disorder. He described feeling anxious about being "monitored" by his family, particularly his sons, who challenged him for being "politically incorrect." He acknowledged some annoyance about this monitoring, though he focused on feeling guilty and worried when he was criticized by them. On some recent occasions, he "unconsciously" drank too much and made unusually inappropriate comments, for which he was reprimanded by his family, leaving him feeling guilty and humiliated. In therapy, it emerged that he was angrier about these "restrictions" than he had been aware of and struggled with the "appropriateness" of these feelings.

MR. Q: I feel ashamed about how I behaved on Sunday, but I realize I don't like my family monitoring me. I shouldn't have to worry about whether I might be saying the wrong thing all the time.

THERAPIST: But I understand that you feel guilty about the comments that you made, that maybe they were too "angry."

MR. Q: I hadn't really thought of it as angry. Maybe "annoyed." But I know my jokes get kind of hostile, especially when I drink.

THERAPIST: It seems like you're in conflict about how angry you get about these restrictions, and you end up trying to manage these feelings by drinking. But drinking causes your irritation to come out even more.

MR. Q: I guess drinking makes me feel like I can express my anger about being monitored, but then I feel terrible afterwards.

THERAPIST: It's important to recognize how angry you are, so you can find ways to help you manage these feelings more effectively.

In exploring his early life, Mr. Q described a bullying father who had intermittent rage episodes, accusing his children of being bad and irresponsible. The therapist worked to link Mr. Q's conflicts over anger to this developmental history, describing his fear and rebellion in response to his father's rages.

THERAPIST: I wonder how much this conflict about anger stems from your reaction to your father's attacks. You experienced them as coming out of the blue and accusing you of all kinds of things you hadn't done. It felt unjust and hurtful, causing you a lot of anxiety, and you didn't dare express anger at him. I wonder if something about being criticized by your sons reminds you of this.

MR. Q: That makes sense. I think it's over the top, like they're always keeping an eye on me. I guess it feels unfair like it did with my father. Also, I don't want to be like him and lose my temper all the time.

THERAPIST: These concerns may interfere with your being able to express normal feelings of frustration and talk to your sons about your feelings.

CASE EXAMPLE: MS. R'S CONFLICT WITH ANGER IN RELATION TO HER MOTHER

Ms. R, a 45-year-old married Black engineer with chronic low self-esteem and recurrent major depression, struggled with any expression of angry feelings. She would enter into relationships, including with her church, in a submissive fashion, volunteering for chores. However, she quickly came to feel that she was not being adequately appreciated for her efforts. In addition, she began to have increasing problems with her husband, and she believed he was behaving in an abusive manner toward her. However, when she addressed her marital problems with the church leaders, she felt they had little sympathy for her.

She was aware of being frustrated but did not make any comments about this to the elders. However, as she became increasingly irritated, she wrote a hostile letter to them describing how hurt she was about them ignoring her. The church leaders were unaware that she had felt angry, and they felt alienated by her letter, eventually suggesting that she leave the church. This triggered severe depression, leading her to seek treatment, in part because she blamed herself for the rejection. The therapist began by more closely examining the triggers of her symptoms.

When the therapist explored with Ms. R why she did not say anything to the church leaders before the letter, she reported fears of expressing any angry feelings. She described how her mother had rages when she was young and often had conflicts with others in the community that led to disruptions in their relationships. In addition, when Ms. R expressed any angry feelings toward her mother, her mother would not speak to her for days. Thus, Ms. R would "stuff down" any anger and continue to feel mistreated until she eventually "blew," having a rage episode similar to her mother's. This led to a surge of intense guilt, shame, and depression.

The therapist linked her fears of expressing anger to anxiety about igniting her mother's wrath and an intense desire to not be like her mother. They began to recognize when she was beginning to get angry about feeling mistreated by others and to see the necessity of addressing these feelings before they developed into a damaging rage. As she understood what made her anger so frightening and the lowered likelihood of problems if she addressed these issues at an earlier point, she became increasingly able to communicate her angry feelings, enabling a negotiation of her frustrations with others.

Conflicts Surrounding Anger Associated with Separation and Dependency Fears

Conflicts about angry feelings are heightened in the setting of separation and dependency fears because of the perceived danger that anger will disrupt needed relationships. These conflicts can lead to normal feelings of ambivalence triggering intense anxiety and guilt, making such feelings difficult to tolerate and effectively manage.

CASE EXAMPLE: MR. Q'S AMBIVALENCE TOWARD HIS WIFE

Mr. Q struggled with mixed feelings about his wife's presence or absence, which sometimes precipitated panic attacks. He often felt frustrated when she was at home and believed that she intruded on his time alone, making demands on him to take care of household chores. However, when monitoring his panic attacks, the therapist and he recognized that they would often occur when his wife would travel for her job. The therapist suggested that, despite his getting annoyed at her intrusiveness, he found it difficult when she was away.

MR. Q: I'm very surprised about that because, when she travels, I'm like "Finally, some time to myself!" But since we've been talking about this, I've noticed that I do feel lonely and anxious when she leaves. I feel more frightened about going out, even though often when she's around I go out by myself without any problem.

THERAPIST: I believe there's something symbolically important about her presence that helps you feel safe. Your father was focused on his work and had terrible temper episodes, and your mother often seemed depressed by his lack of attention. Seems like you often felt left alone emotionally.

MR. Q: Yeah. I'd sometimes play games with my sister, but it could be pretty lonely in the house. And I often felt pressure to take care of my mother, who seemed pretty down. So, it was tough finding a safe spot.

THERAPIST: And that seems to be the case now, as you feel either too controlled or too lonely. These feelings seem to be in conflict but actually represent two ways of experiencing yourself with others that can feel very unsafe.

MR. Q: I guess I don't like to acknowledge that I need her because then I might allow her to try to control me. It's a real "push/pull" I guess.

CASE EXAMPLE: MS. G'S PEOPLE PLEASING

Ms. G, discussed in Chapter 2 as struggling with anxiety symptoms, referred to herself as a "people pleaser." She described, for example, a friend of hers, Lucinda, who tended to take advantage of her by asking her to give advice about her relationships with men, but then spent little time socially with her, or would drop plans with her to meet other friends. She began to recognize what she described as Lucinda's "user" behavior, but she denied being angry with her. She felt badly that Lucinda had such difficult problems with boyfriends, which Ms. G patiently helped her with. However, as she proceeded in her treatment, Ms. G began to feel that Lucinda took advantage of her and that her friend's behavior was unfair. The therapist inquired whether she would ever consider talking to Lucinda about these matters:

Ms. G: Oh, no. I don't think I could possibly do that.

THERAPIST: What would your concerns be?

Ms. G: I guess I haven't said much about it, but Lucinda has dropped friends and boyfriends in a second, particularly if they confront her about some problem.

THERAPIST: Have you considered whether you want to be friends with someone like that?

Ms. G: I've started to wonder about it. I'm not sure what I'm really getting out of the relationship. But I don't want her to be mad at me. I'd be really upset.

THERAPIST: Do you feel mad at her?

Ms. G: I just feel badly for her. Although lately I have felt more frustrated.

THERAPIST: I know you're worried about her dropping you as a friend, but it doesn't seem like you're getting much out of the relationship.

Ms. G: That's a good point. I'll have to think about it. Maybe it doesn't make sense to try so hard. But I get worried that if she gets mad, I won't have any friends left. Although I realize that's not true.

The dialogue above describes how the therapist worked both to elucidate the patient's conflict and reduce the catastrophic fears associated with it. Additionally, the therapist identified how this conflict was triggering problems in her relationships.

CASE EXAMPLE: MS. S'S PANIC ATTACKS

Ms. S, a 36-year-old married White laboratory technician, suffered from panic attacks that therapeutic exploration found to be related to conflicts surrounding anger and fears of separation or disruption. These attacks would occur in circumstances where she felt devalued, not recognized for her abilities, or criticized and harshly judged. Triggers of these feelings included get-togethers with her brother and father and at work.

In these situations, Ms. S described feeling trapped and hopeless, unable to extract herself from the problematic situation she was in. For example, she felt left out when her father and brother discussed their jobs in sales, which the patient had little interest in, as she worked in medical research. At work, she felt that her contributions were minimized, in part because she was a woman, and she believed that men who were academically promoted had fewer capabilities than she did.

THERAPIST: Do you get angry about how you're treated?

MS. S: I do feel frustrated, but mostly I feel anxious and trapped.

THERAPIST: Have you ever expressed your frustration about this to your father or boss?

MS. S: I don't think that would go over very well with them. My father had a terrible temper when we were young, and he doesn't respond very well to somebody disagreeing with him, especially if he thinks they're being critical. And my boss, if someone complains to him, he's been known to fire them.

THERAPIST: So how do you manage your anger?

MS. S: I really try to push it out of my mind because I don't want to end up alone or lose my job. When my father gets mad, he becomes harsh and very difficult to be around.

THERAPIST: You do seem to feel a very high threat in expressing your frustration based on your father's behavior. I think it would be important to further address these fears and see if you might be overestimating the risks with others because this approach creates a lot of frustration and anxiety for you.

Conflicts with Autonomy and Separation Fears

Separation fears often intensify a sense of dependency on others, creating a potential area of conflict. These fears are prominent in patients with insecure attachment or fearful dependency on others. Conflicts can occur between wishes for autonomy and the potential dangers of separation this can create.

CASE EXAMPLE: MS. T'S AUTONOMY FEARS

Ms. T, a 32-year-old White graduate student, developed the onset of intense panic while working on her thesis, becoming unable to focus. This panic did not occur when Ms. T was reading material unrelated to her graduate work. Although she went to college in another city, Ms. T moved back to live with her mother for graduate school. Her mother took care of the cooking, cleaning, and laundry, despite her mother working a full-time job. Nevertheless, Ms. T would fight with her about intruding into the patient's room to clean (mother claimed the room became unsanitary) and then experience intense guilt, fearing her mother would die.

Ms. T's history was notable for the sudden death of her father at age 3. It emerged that Ms. T feared the loss of her mother if she were to move forward with grad school and become independent. Although she reported no memory of her father, the fears of loss of her mother appeared to have derived from his sudden death and the ongoing impact this had on her mother in terms of depressive symptoms through the course of her childhood. This awareness helped to better address her fears of autonomy, as they were derived from past traumatic experiences rather than actual completion of graduate school.

Conflicts Surrounding Dependency on Others

Dependency fears are particularly intensified with patients who have early life disruptions with caregivers. These experiences can increase both longings to be taken care of and fears that patients will be rejected or abandoned. The link to distressing early life experiences can often be useful in recognizing and addressing these conflicts.

CASE EXAMPLE: MS. U'S CONFLICTS WITH DEPENDENCY

Ms. U was a 48-year-old married Black female who, with the agreement of her husband, quit her job as an administrative assistant to pursue her passion for writing. Despite the opportunity to follow her interest, she developed the onset of generalized anxiety and moderate depressive symptoms. As she began treatment, it emerged that she felt increasingly fearfully dependent on her husband Richard for financial support. Exploration revealed that she feared Richard would reject her, as her previous husband had done, for being too "dependent" on him. The therapist reminded her of Richard's reassurance that he did not mind taking care of her financially, leading to some relief of her symptoms.

In exploring her early life, Ms. U, who was the youngest of four siblings, described significant time at home alone with her mother. Her mother drank daily, which worsened over the years, and became critical and abusive toward the patient when she did so. She yelled that Ms. U was unwanted and had created a burden for her that greatly limited her lifestyle and had thought about how to "get rid of her." Ms. U felt frightened and guilty in the face of her mother's attacks on her, as well as worried about her mother's safety. On a few occasions, her father would come home and find her mother asleep, yelling at both his wife and the patient for creating this situation. Thus, the therapist was able to further link her dependency fears to her childhood experience. Indeed, even as she chose her husband on the basis of his being caring toward her and "very unlike my parents," she was worried that he would shift his attitude and want to "get rid of her" as she became more financially dependent.

Conflicts about Sexual Wishes

Sexual fantasies are a common source of conflict, particularly if these wishes are associated with aggressive or dependent feelings. Helping patients understand the origins of such wishes can help them to reduce the anxiety and guilt they create.

CASE EXAMPLE: MR. V'S DISTRESSING SEXUAL FANTASIES

Mr. V, a 62-year-old single White artist, reported chronic conflict about sexual fantasies of forcing women to yield to him, which triggered intense guilty feelings, along with persistent anxiety and depression. Mr. V reported extensive abuse and trauma as a child. His brother was verbally and physically abusive, and his parents were slow to intervene. He was particularly terrified of being left alone with his brother, when there appeared to be no limits on his verbal and physical attacks. His mother had recurrent depressive episodes, sometimes with psychotic elements. His father was critical and rejecting of the patient. He found his son's interest in dance and art to be "effeminate" and said he "wouldn't amount to anything."

He felt terribly embarrassed when he revealed more details about these fantasies:

MR. V: I've been troubled for years by these violent sexual fantasies. I mean I would never act on them, but I can't believe I have them in the first place. I really don't want to tell you about them because I'm convinced you'll think very negatively about me.

THERAPIST: It sounds like it would be important for you to tell me about them. Of course, people have a very wide range of sexual fantasies, but these seem to cause you tremendous pain and guilt.

MR. V: Yes, I find them exciting but then I really suffer about having them. In them, I force people to do what I want sexually, but then they really enjoy it. It's hard to say more.

THERAPIST: More details would likely help me understand them better, but for right now, I wonder how much these fantasies relate to the hurt and pain your brother caused you. It's as if somehow you've turned these fantasies around and you're doing them to others. You're the one in control.

MR. V: I hadn't really thought of them that way. But then why are they sexual fantasies? Why not fantasies about beating someone else up? I mean I guess I do have some of those, too.

THERAPIST: It's not unusual for other feelings to get caught up in sexual fantasies. So, aggression can show up sexually, although it's obviously important that you've never acted on it. And the fantasies show another reversal in that the other person ends up enjoying it, as opposed to the hurt and pain you felt with your brother.

MR. V: I see what you're saying, though I still really struggle with having them in the first place. All these years I thought I was just a terrible person.

CASE EXAMPLE: MR. W'S CONFLICTED SEXUAL FANTASIES ABOUT MEN

Mr. W, a 52-year-old divorced White man who worked in finance, was highly conflicted about sexual fantasies involving muscular men who admired him for being powerful and therefore wanted to have sex with him. He was very embarrassed about these fantasies and believed that they meant he was "unmanly." Mr. W reported a history of significant bullying by his father, who criticized and attacked others who disagreed with his views or actions. For example, when Mr. W expressed interest in going to drama camp, his father refused to allow this, calling Mr. W a "wimp." His father was friendlier to his older brother, who was "all boy."

Mr. W emphasized to the therapist that, despite these fantasies, he was not interested in having sex with men and was attracted to women. The therapist reassured Mr. W that people had all kinds of sexual fantasies and could certainly have them involving both sexes. In addition, the therapist noted that these sexual fantasies had several meanings that were important for the patient and compensatory for the problems he had in the relationship with his father. For example, he was admired rather than demeaned, dominating rather than bullied, and intensely close to a man rather than distant, as he felt with his father. This understanding significantly eased Mr. W's conflict about these fantasies and helped him better recognize how he attempted to cope with the adverse events of his childhood.

DEFENSES

Defense mechanisms (see Chapter 1) represent the ways in which patients characteristically attempt to cope with distressing emotions, negative self and other representations, and/or conflicted feelings and fantasies (A. Freud, 1936). Defenses typically operate outside of conscious awareness, and an important therapeutic task is helping patients become aware of the presence and function of these defenses. Upon identifying these defenses, therapists can better access and address the conflicted feelings and fantasies that trigger them. Some ways of handling difficult feelings are considered more adaptive and operate consciously, such as **humor** and **suppression**. In using suppression, the individual consciously sets aside painful feelings, fantasies, or experiences.

Several defenses play a role in attempting to manage angry feelings and fantasies that are a source of conflict. These include **reaction formation**, in which the individual adopts a compensatory submissiveness or caretaking of others toward whom they are actually angry. In the defense of **undoing**, individuals symbolically or verbally take back an angry expression or wish. They might be heard saying of a partner, "I despise him, but I really love him." While such defenses can be found normally or in any disorder, they are common in panic and other anxiety disorders, in which the individual is attempting to manage anger and make their attachment feel more secure. In the defense of **passive**

aggression, individuals express anger indirectly via behaviors such as lateness and withholding.

Ms. G demonstrated the use of **reaction formation** in her relationship with Lucinda, described above. Despite her disappointment at Lucinda only getting together with her when she needed her help, while socializing with other friends, she felt upset about Lucinda's troubles with men and that it was important to help her deal with these feelings. Thus, she was willing to accept spending time with Lucinda to talk through her troubles. As she began to comprehend the pressure she felt to respond to others' needs and how it contributed to her anxiety, she increasingly recognized the anger she felt at others who were not recognizing her needs. She was able to identify her anger at Lucinda, and the pressure to take care of her when she was upset eased. Although she did not directly confront Lucinda, she increasingly set limits on getting together just to discuss her problems, insisting on a social activity instead. Lucinda was responsive to these efforts, leading to the reduction of Ms. G's anger and use of reaction formation.

Repression is a defense mechanism through which feelings, fantasies, and memories that create conflict, pain, and anxiety are kept from conscious awareness. In dealing with repression, the therapist works to bring emotions, thoughts, and memories to consciousness by helping patients become aware of and feel safer with these mental states. An associated defense, **denial**, also operates to keep painful feelings and fantasies out of awareness. **Projection** is a defense in which anger is denied and experienced as coming from someone else rather than the individual expressing it. Anger at others can also be **directed toward the self**.

Other defenses function to ward off low self-esteem. Individuals can counter feelings of inadequacy by **idealizing** aspects of themselves or others with whom they are emotionally connected. This is a common dynamic in patients with narcissistic personality and depressive disorders, in which compensatory idealization can lead to significant disappointment for patients in themselves and others when they are unable to meet expectations. People may also work to prop up their self-esteem by emphasizing the negative traits of others, using the defense of **devaluation**.

For example, further therapeutic work with Ms. R indicated that she used the defenses of idealization, reaction formation, passive aggression, and projection in efforts to manage her anger. After her problems with the church, Ms. R had an improvement in her symptoms when she joined a volunteer organization that aided immigrants, whose leaders she idealized, viewing them as people who deeply cared about others (**idealization**). Her feelings of chronic inadequacy and low self-esteem experienced a boost from being accepted by this group. As part of her usual pattern, she began to do extensive tasks for the organization, including cleaning and cooking at volunteer events. However, over time she started to become upset that her efforts were not recognized and that she was not asked to do more direct work with helping immigrants. In addition, she started to observe significant tensions within the group and even some mistreatment of the immigrants they were supposed to be helping.

Ms. R experienced increasing disappointment and anger with the leaders but continued to struggle with how to express those feelings. She began to do her chores halfheartedly, or sometimes even forget to complete them, while sulking in the presence of others (**passive aggression**). Rather than asking what troubled her, the organization's leaders criticized her for backing off on these tasks. This led to a further surge in her anger, but she felt terribly guilty, as she believed she was letting down the organization. Her feelings of inadequacy returned, and she blamed herself for her lack of motivation (**anger directed inward**). She began to believe that the group's leaders wanted nothing to do with her because of her inadequacies (**projection**), although other than the reprimand about chores, they remained friendly toward her. She redoubled her efforts to take care of tasks because she felt concerned that the group's leaders were overwhelmed (**reaction formation**) and these efforts would earn her the hoped-for praise.

In the above example, Ms. R demonstrated the use of several defense mechanisms to manage her conflict regarding her feelings of inadequacy, disappointment, and anger with the volunteer group leaders. At first, she **idealized** the organization's leaders in an effort to relieve her low self-esteem. However, as often occurs with this defense, she became disappointed with their lack of responsiveness and infighting. Rather than expressing her frustration directly, she responded first with **passive aggression**, failing to complete tasks she had agreed to and sulking. Additionally, she directed her anger toward herself, blaming herself for the lack of motivation. She shifted to the use of **projection**, believing that the organization's leaders were angry at her because she was behaving badly. Finally, she demonstrated the use of **reaction formation**, suppressing her anger and escalating her efforts to support the group leaders, which she believed would earn their love and admiration. As the therapist brought these various defenses to her attention, they were able to more directly address her struggles with feelings of inadequacy and anger and address the problems with the organization. As opposed to what had happened with her church, she was able to resolve her tensions with the leaders and continue working with the group.

Somatization is a defense in which impulses and fantasies that are experienced as dangerous are displaced onto the body or worries about one's health. This defense is seen prominently in a number of disorders, including anxiety, panic, and depression.

Ms. S, described previously, reported panic attacks with palpitations that occurred when she felt frustrated by men whom she described as mean and disregarding, especially her boss:

THERAPIST: So, you notice that you feel increased stress and palpitations when your boss is critical of you?

MS. S: Yes, and he doesn't really know what he's doing. He's judging me when he has no idea of the work involved in this technical area.

THERAPIST: Are you aware of feeling angry at him?

Ms. S: Yes, but my focus really switches to my anxiety, and then I start worrying about my body. My heart starts racing, and I worry there's something wrong with my heart. That's when I really start to panic.

Therapist: Would you be worried about getting angry with him?

Ms. S: I don't think I could get angry. He's so thin-skinned that I don't know what he'd do. He might fire me. But as we talk about it, you know what makes me really angry? He's not recognizing my skill set and acting like I'm incompetent. And he's really the one who's incompetent. But even as I think about that now, I'm starting to get anxious, and my heart is speeding up.

Therapist: What do you think is going on?

Ms. S: I don't know. Maybe it really is scary getting angry at him.

Therapist: I think anxiety about your anger gets displaced onto your body. Even though that's frightening, I think it's less dangerous to you than what you believe will happen if you express your anger.

Fears of loss of control of feelings and impulses can be displaced to fears of loss of control of the body; this could be seen in Ms. S's worry that her heart was in danger when she also feared her anger was out of control. Indeed, exploration of her background revealed a father who was highly temperamental and had difficulty tolerating any "noise" from his children, such as she and her brother arguing or even play fighting. Somatic symptoms can also derive from a lack of capacity to identify bodily aspects of emotions, such as those that can be part of anxiety and anger. Thus, Ms. S's racing heart could be understood as a component of her anger and anxiety that could not be recognized, as she saw it more as a problem with her body.

In the defense of **dissociation**, a disruption occurs in the normally integrated thoughts, feelings, memories, consciousness, and identity. For example, an individual may describe a traumatic event while experiencing an absence of emotion or sense of numbness. Alternatively, individuals can experience anxious or depressive symptoms clearly related to trauma but not consciously make the connection. Dissociation often functions as a defense against painful memories and emotions associated with traumatic experiences. Pervasive numbing can be another form of dissociation that avoids the distress associated with the trauma or the experience of profound loss or guilt.

Splitting represents a defense often found in borderline personality disorder or those exposed to severe trauma. In this defense, the individual unconsciously protects others from his or her rage by separating "all good" from "all bad" others, who are deserving of contempt and aggression. These black-and-white perceptions are typically dissociated, interfering with the capacity of the individual to integrate them. One outcome of this defense is sudden shifts from highly positive to highly negative perceptions of others and associated mood lability. Poor impulse control often results from these intense affects.

CASE EXAMPLE: MS. X'S SHIFT BETWEEN "ALL GOOD" AND "ALL BAD"

Ms. X, a 50-year-old divorced lawyer, reported recurrent severe depressive episodes, brief and easily disrupted relationships, episodes of rage and mood lability, fears of abandonment, impulsivity, and thoughts of suicide, consistent with a diagnosis of borderline personality disorder. She felt alone and angry, believing that her friends had not adequately supported her during her divorce, and had ended these relationships. She was unemployed, having lost interest in her legal career, and was uncertain what new area to pursue.

Her involvement with her family left her feeling down, anxious, and frustrated. She viewed her mother as controlling and exploiting others, but after visiting home, she shifted to seeing her as a helpless victim of her alcoholic father's abusive behavior. When she saw her mother as victimized, she felt guilty and pressured to "rescue" her. But after leaving the home environment, she became furious that her mother would do nothing to change her situation. She also felt depressed and enraged by her father's attacks on her, calling her "crazy" and "disappointing."

In reviewing her pattern in relationships, the therapist noted how she would initially view others as supportive but ultimately shift to a sense that they were uncaring and self-focused. Ms. X would then castigate herself for not having recognized at an earlier point how damaging these others were. When, prior to a visit home, she shifted to the view of her mother as victimized, the therapist noted how she typically ended up feeling enraged and exploited. At this point, her rage shifted toward the therapist, attacking him for not recognizing her mother's need for help, providing an opportunity to identify these "good to bad" shifts in the transference.

MS. X: I can't believe you don't understand why I need to go to my mother's to help her. I feel like I should quit treatment.

THERAPIST: I think the same pattern is happening with me as with others. You find me helpful, but then subsequently you feel angry and disappointed.

MS. X: We've talked about that pattern, but I just feel that right now you don't get me and don't think therapy is helping.

THERAPIST: I think it's important that you see how much your feelings can shift, to help better manage your anger and disappointment.

MS. X: I'll consider what you're saying. I feel like you're not helping now, but I know I've felt differently before.

In between the stormy periods, Ms. X became more willing to explore how her feelings changed. She increasingly recognized how her polarized view of others and herself led to a surge in anger and disappointment that hurt herself and her relationships.

Mr. Q's drinking behavior was an example of the defense of **acting out**. He was conflicted about his angry feelings toward what he viewed as "monitoring" and expressed his anger indirectly by drinking, which was upsetting to his family. Reducing his drinking helped him find new ways of managing his anger.

In the defense of **identification with the aggressor**, patients connect their own self-image with an aggressive individual, particularly someone who had power over them. Mr. W, described previously, who felt bullied by his father throughout his childhood and beyond, would at times shift to bullying others. Exploration revealed that this bullying would lead him to feel power and control, the opposite of what he felt with his father. Thus, he demonstrated the defense of identification with the aggressor, connecting his self-image with that of his father, dominating and pressuring others. However, after acting on these behaviors, he would often experience a surge in guilty feelings for attacking others the way he was attacked. In another example of this defense, Mr. V's violent sexual fantasies involved taking control over others, as his brother did with him.

Although defenses mostly operate out of awareness, certain probes can give preliminary information about patients' propensity to these defenses (described below but also available online as Worksheet 5.2: How You Manage Your Feelings and Wishes, pp. 130–132). In the session, you might explain to your patient that it will shed light on their problems to get more specific about how they manage feelings or wishes, which may cause them discomfort or feel threatening. You can use the questions presented as a guide for your clinical interview, or you can give them the worksheet, saying, "In the next few days, before our next session, I'd like you to try completing this worksheet. It asks you to try describing how you manage your feelings and wishes." Their responses can then be used as a basis for further exploration of their defenses.

> **Reaction formation:** Do you find that, when someone makes you angry, you're more likely to respond by being nice or wanting to take care of them?
>
> **Undoing:** Do you find that you deny or take back your angry or vengeful feelings when you have or express them?
>
> **Passive aggression:** When you get angry at someone, do you sometimes express it by being late to meetings or slowing down work on tasks you're supposed to do for them?
>
> **Denial/repression:** Do you believe that you don't get angry at other people?
>
> **Idealization:** Do you seek out the best of everything, including the best people?
>
> **Devaluation:** Do you sometimes put down others to make yourself feel better?
>
> **Splitting:** Do you tend to see others as either good or bad and not much in between?
>
> **Somatization:** Have you noticed any connection between bodily feelings that you're

having and stress that you're experiencing? When you get angry, do you feel like something is going wrong with your body?

Acting out: When you're angry, do you act on those feelings—for example, by verbally or physically attacking or bullying someone? By drinking?

Self-directed anger: Do you notice that, after you get angry at someone, you tend to get angry at yourself or criticize yourself for feeling angry?

Suppression: When you get angry, do you notice you tend to push these feelings aside or try not to think about them?

Humor: When you get angry do you look for ways to joke around about it?

COMPROMISE FORMATION

A compromise formation (see Chapter 1) is a mental state and/or behavior that involves a conflicted wish, guilt or anxiety about the wish, and a defense against the wish. The compromise, which can be a symptom, often contains a partial but disguised fulfillment of the wish and a defense against the consequences of that wish. Below are described examples of compromise formation from cases discussed previously.

In her overspending, Ms. J (see Chapters 2 and 3) unconsciously expressed her anger about the limits that her husband was trying to set with her financially and obtained something that she experienced as taken away from her, in having felt abandoned by her mother. The wish that was most conflicted was needing something from others, as she had attempted to minimize the impact of her mother's behavior, believing that she could manage things on her own. As these wishes emerged into consciousness in therapy, she recognized the degree of deprivation and anger that she felt toward her mother, who left the home when the patient was 12 years old, leaving the patient, her brother, and father with limited financial and emotional support. She began to recognize feeling deprived and angry, which helped her better manage these feelings, avoiding expressing them through impulse shopping.

Mr. F's overworking both yielded to his father's demands about not being a "loser" and rebelled against them by not focusing fully on his clients while worrying that he would get caught doing this. He also expressed his anger at feeling devalued by his family indirectly by avoiding time with them. Untangling these elements of "compromise" helped him better manage his workaholic behavior.

Mr. Q's drinking represented an indirect expression of his anger about "policing" and enabled him to make "edgier" comments. Thus, he rebelled against his father's strictures and arranged punishment from his family via reprimand, triggering a wave of guilt and shame. Untangling these factors that contributed to his acting out helped him to more directly identify and address his anger.

In the context of formulating self and other representations and conflicts and defenses, with a goal of addressing contributors to problems, the therapist also works with patients to improve mentalization skills. This capacity to identify mental states in self and others, discussed in Chapter 6, is another important factor in addressing problems.

> **QUESTIONS AND IDEAS TO THINK ABOUT**
>
> 1. With one of your current patients, try identifying their predominant intrapsychic conflicts. What interventions do you think would be able to address these?
> 2. With one of your current patients, try identifying their predominant defenses. What might be useful ways to bring these to the patient's attention and begin to determine what triggers them?

WORKSHEET 5.1
Conflicts about Feelings and Fantasies

These questions will help you and your therapist gather information about and address your problems by getting more detail about feelings or wishes that you are conflicted about.

Are you aware of any problems you have with angry feelings or expressing your anger?

Do you have fears about depending on other people?

Do you have fears about other people depending on you?

(continued)

From *Skills Training in Psychodynamic Psychotherapy*, by Fredric N. Busch. Copyright © 2026 The Guilford Press. Permission to photocopy this worksheet, or to download and print additional copies (*www.guilford.com/busch-forms*), is granted to purchasers of this book for personal use or use with clients; see copyright page for details.

Conflicts about Feelings and Fantasies *(page 2 of 2)*

Do you have fears about separating from others?

Do you struggle with mixed feelings about others?

Are there any difficulties you have with your sexual feelings and fantasies?

WORKSHEET 5.2

How You Manage Your Feelings and Wishes

These questions will help you and your therapist gather information about and address your problems by getting more detail about how you manage feelings or wishes.

Do you find that, when someone makes you angry, you're more likely to respond by being nice or wanting to take care of them?

Do you find that you deny or take back your angry or vengeful feelings when you have or express them?

When you get angry at someone, do you sometimes express it by being late to meetings or slowing down work on tasks you're supposed to do for them?

Do you believe that you don't get angry at other people?

(continued)

How You Manage Your Feelings and Wishes (page 2 of 3)

Do you seek out the best of everything, including the best people?

Do you sometimes put down others to make yourself feel better?

Do you tend to see others as either good or bad and not much in between?

Have you noticed any connection between bodily feelings that you're having and stress that you're experiencing? When you get angry, do you feel like something is going wrong with your body?

(continued)

How You Manage Your Feelings and Wishes *(page 3 of 3)*

When you're angry, do you act on those feelings—for example, by verbally or physically attacking or bullying someone? By drinking?

Do you notice that, after you get angry at someone, you tend to get angry at yourself or criticize yourself for feeling angry?

When you get angry, do you notice that you tend to push these feelings aside or try not to think about them?

When you get angry, do you look for ways to joke around about it?

CHAPTER 6

Developing Mentalization Skills

This chapter focuses on the development of mentalization skills, the capacity to consider what is happening in one's own mind and the minds of others (Fonagy, 2008). Self-reflection, already a focus of the book, is discussed, but mentalization skills also include thinking about what might be influencing others to behave the way they do. These skills can be used to reduce the tendency toward blaming oneself for others' reactions and to better understand how to negotiate one's needs with others. A worksheet provides a means of practicing thinking about the mental states of self and others and consider the implications of this information with regard to problem solving. Case examples demonstrate working with patients to improve mentalization skills and diminish a variety of problems.

CASE EXAMPLE: MS. Y'S WORRIES ABOUT "RETIREMENT"

Ms. Y, a 52-year-old White laboratory researcher who struggled with anxious and depressive symptoms in part related to job stress, was uncomfortable about telling people that she had taken a leave from her job for 3 months and was considering not returning to it. She viewed this as an important step toward pursuing her own goals and wishes, as opposed to a job that she had felt pressured to do by her family, which had several scientists in it. She was worried that others might be judgmental toward her, viewing her as lazy or as having "retired." Ms. Y did not see this action as either quitting work or retiring, but instead as taking time to pursue other interests. However, when she did tell others about her situation, some seem puzzled or indeed appeared judgmental, saying things such as, "Well, why aren't you working?" or "What are you going to do without a job?" This kind of response would lead to waves of feeling badly and criticizing her own decision.

The therapist had explored Ms. Y's vulnerability in self-esteem that led her to be easily injured by these comments, and Ms. Y had been making efforts to recognize these factors. The tools she developed from gaining these understandings included identifying how her overreaction was based on her mother's harsh judgments toward her and her tendency to direct that criticism toward herself. At this point, the therapist pursued the patient's use of mentalization skills to consider why others might be reacting in the way they did. The therapist explored with her what others might be experiencing when they appeared to be critical:

THERAPIST: I think you're overly concerned about others being judgmental, as it's important for you to take this step, but to the extent that they are, I wonder what you think might be going on with them?

MS. Y: I really hadn't thought about that.

THERAPIST: One idea I had is that perhaps what makes them uncomfortable is that they're working, and they're not used to the idea of someone suddenly stopping a job.

MS. Y: That makes some sense. I guess it's also possible that they may be jealous or thinking, "She's lucky she has the money to not work." Which I really don't, but I am able to stop working for a while.

THERAPIST: That's an important thought about jealousy. We know you're pursuing doing what you want to do. But with your mother, that wasn't okay. She would attack you for pursuing what you wanted because it wasn't what she wanted you to do or because she was jealous.

MS. Y: That's true. And if I think about it, what was the reason she was judgmental? I wonder if she was envious of my going after what I wanted—something she never did herself. I mean, what was it to her, or to anybody now, if I'm working or not?"

THERAPIST: It's a good question. And important to consider when you suddenly start feeling bad and start chastising yourself for taking a break.

Encouraging Ms. Y to use her mentalization skills eased her self-critical reactions to others' negative comments about her taking a break from work, which she expected based on her developmental experiences and self and other representations.

EXPLORING MENTALIZATION SKILLS

Below are some questions that patients can consider using to enhance their mentalization skills. (A worksheet with these questions, Worksheet 6.1: Understanding What Is

Happening in Your Own and Others' Minds, pp. 149–150, as well as all other worksheets, is available at *www.guilford.com/busch-forms*). In the session, you might explain to patients that these questions will help them think about what is going on in their own mind and the minds of others. You can use the questions presented as a guide for your clinical interview, or you can give them the worksheet, saying, "In the next few days, before our next session, I'd like you to try completing this worksheet. It asks you to try describing what is going on in your own mind and the minds of others as it relates to your problems." The responses can then be used to discuss and further develop mentalization skills. Below are Ms. Y's responses to these questions:

Describe the problems you have with one of your relationships and your feelings about it.

When I told my friend Joan I was taking a few months off to consider what I want to do, she seemed critical of that step. She said, "How are you going to afford not working?" I didn't feel I had to answer, but then I felt badly, thinking, "Am I doing the right thing?"

Consider the feelings and problems you are having with someone from the other person's perspective, imagining the responses the other person might have.

I guess Joan could be jealous. She feels stuck in her job, and I bet she would want to take off time if she could.

How do you understand the differences in perspective you have with the other person regarding the problem in the relationship?

I feel that I'm taking this big, important step in my life, and she kind of poured cold water on it. Then I became self-critical about it. But now I have a better idea why.

If someone is criticizing or judging you, what do you think might lead that person to react the way they do? Pick a specific instance or two to consider.

I had another instance where my friend Jillian also reacted kind of weirdly. She said, "Oh. Are you retiring? What are you going to do with your time? Watch TV?" I thought it was kind of a mean reaction, thinking I would just be lazy. It does seem like people have a hard time with this information.

When that person criticized you, how much did it have to do with you, and what might be going on with the other person?

I think this has more to do with her. I know she's a really hard worker, and I think it would be tough for her to consider the possibility that someone else could just not work. She would probably think it's lazy. But I know I'm also sensitive about criticism.

In a recent conflict you had with someone, what do you think that person might have been reacting to?

I got mad at my husband for watching TV and not doing the chores. But now I'm thinking maybe I'm focused on that because I felt guilty about stopping work, and I didn't think he should be "lazy." I know he had a stressful week and should probably give him a break. Though sometimes he does drag his feet on the chores, and that's annoying.

When Ms. Y brought her responses to the next session, the therapist reviewed them with her to further improve her mentalizing skills. The therapist noted in the last response on the worksheet how the patient used these skills to both better understand what was going on with her husband and with herself in the conflict they were having. This awareness helped diminish the tension between them.

CASE EXAMPLE: MS. Z'S INTENSE GUILT

Ms. Z, a 68-year-old Latina former realtor had retired and planned to devote herself full time to her writing. Problems that brought her to treatment included fears of exposing her creative work to others, out of concern that they would be critical of it. However, another problem had emerged since retirement with her daughter Valerie, who expected Ms. Z to spend significant portions of her time taking care of her grandson. Ms. Z wanted to be available for babysitting but did not want to be a "full-time" grandmother. In addition, there were recurrent problems with her daughter, a single mother whom the patient often financially supported.

Despite this support, Valerie was often critical of her, complaining that Ms. Z was an absent mother and had "abandoned" her as a child. While indeed she did have to work when her daughter was very young, Ms. Z believed that Valerie's view of abandonment was greatly exaggerated. Nevertheless, Ms. Z struggled with guilt about wanting time to herself, and Valerie's accusations deepened her guilty feelings. Actually, Valerie had experienced abandonment with her father, who spent lengthy periods away on business and ultimately had an affair that led to divorce. After the divorce, Ms. Z's ex-husband had minimal contact with Valerie, although she rarely expressed frustration with him.

In exploring her early development, Ms. Z described her mother as having had a drinking problem that often required her and her younger brother to intervene, as her father was frequently away on business. Despite these factors, her mother often complained that Ms. Z did not pay enough attention to her, which likely related to feelings of abandonment by her husband. Ms. Z's father did little to address her mother's drinking when he was present, shutting himself in his room to work. Despite these problems inappropriately falling on her, Ms. Z felt guilty that she could not do more for her mother and that her mother was dissatisfied with her. Some of these problems appeared to be recapitulated with her daughter.

The therapist and Ms. Z had been exploring her proneness toward guilt based on her developmental experiences, and he believed it would be useful to encourage the patient's use of mentalization skills:

Ms. Z: I really want to have my time to myself, but when Valerie starts complaining about my not being there when she was a child, my guilt really kicks in. Then I agree to spend more time there. After that, I feel frustrated because I want my own life! I don't have time to work on my writing.

THERAPIST: We want to look at your guilt because you've said that your daughter's complaints are very much overstated. We know that you're prone to feeling guilty based on the pressure you felt to take care of your own mother.

Ms. Z: That's true and I try to keep that in mind when I start to feel guilty and pressured to spend more time with her. Then I get mad that I agreed to it.

THERAPIST: We also know that you believe your daughter exaggerates the degree to which you deprived her. This sounds reminiscent of your mother's inappropriate expectations of caretaking with regard to her drinking.

Ms. Z: I see what you're saying. My daughter and I had a fight the other day. She was saying that she never had a home-cooked meal because I was exhausted and distracted when I got home from work. But that's not true. I frequently stopped at the grocery store and cooked for her. She said that wasn't what happened. Maybe it's a small point, but it's related to her whole attitude. And you know what? She still doesn't say anything about her father not being home.

THERAPIST: What do you think of that?

Ms. Z: It makes no sense. If anyone was depriving, he was.

THERAPIST: Have you spoken to her about this?

Ms. Z: I can't really. If I do, she gets really angry. She says, "You're always blaming him."

THERAPIST: It sounds tough. We should consider your going into family therapy to address these problems with her. However, I think you're realizing that this denial of her father's role is important. It sounds like you're saying she displaces anger at her father toward you. Kind of like your mother displaced her anger at your father toward you.

Ms. Z: It definitely seems that way. Maybe because the few times he saw her he was nice? I mean he can be charming and generous, but he had almost nothing to do with her. He was very focused on his new family.

THERAPIST: It seems like your understanding of this could help you with the guilt that you feel. You reflexively react when she starts blaming you for having deprived her, but recognizing that this isn't a fair assessment can help you challenge that guilt. Hopefully, that could help you from going into this cycle of guilt, doing too much, and then feeling angry with her.

Ms. Z: It's a good point. It doesn't make sense that I feel so guilty and pressured based on needing to make up for something from her childhood. I know I had issues as a mom, but I wasn't abandoning in the way she claims.

Over time, using her mentalization skills and understanding the impact of developmental contributors helped ease Ms. Z's intense guilt about her daughter. She realized that this guilt led her to overly solicitous behavior and an inability to set boundaries to maintain her writing. In the weeks that followed, she was able to make clear to her daughter that she needed some time to spend on her work but had no intention of being abandoning. They were able to agree to stretches of time when she could be by herself to focus on her art.

Mentalization Skills in Dealing with Children

Ms. Z's developing mentalization skills also needed to be put to use in addressing issues with her grandson. Indeed, mentalization skills are highly important for parents to use in addressing the behavior and attitudes of their children (Slade et al., 2023). For instance, some parents will misinterpret a child's temper tantrum as a deliberate effort to upset the life of the parent, saying, for example, "He's just being a jerk." Their anger at the child only tends to exacerbate the child's frustration. In these instances, it is important that the parent begin to recognize that the child is most likely hungry, tired, or needing more attention from the parent. Mentalization interventions (Slade et al., 2023) have been shown to be highly effective at addressing such problems.

Rather than misinterpreting her grandson's negative behavior, Ms. Z's problem was that her grandson's expression of longings for her only exacerbated the guilt she felt about separating from her daughter. When Ms. Z had spent time away from her daughter and grandson, and again pursued her own interests, she would frequently speak with her grandson on video. At one point, he expressed his feelings about her being away:

Ms. Z: He said, "I miss you, grandma." And when he said that, my heart just broke. I felt again like I should drop everything and go there.

Therapist: It sounds like he's just expressing a wish to be with you—a natural response to your separation.

Ms. Z: I get that. But I didn't even know a 2-year-old was able to express it that way.

Therapist: How did you interpret what he was saying?

Ms. Z: I felt it meant he must be having a miserable time there with his mother, and he was really hoping I'd come back to relieve that situation.

Therapist: That sounds like an overinterpretation based on your guilt, or maybe your own longings to be with him. It sounds like he misses you and wishes you were around, and he's very good at expressing his feelings. However, he didn't say anything about being miserable or upset with his mom, did he?

Ms. Z: No, but he has entered his terrible twos stage, and he fights more with his mom. And she doesn't like that. She sees him as just being bad.

THERAPIST: It sounds like it would be good for you to explain to her that 2-year-olds are just going to push boundaries. That's part of who they are. He's not trying to create trouble. But your idea that you just need to drop everything and go there because he expressed these feelings seems like a problem. Obviously, you want to be available to help, but you also want to pursue your own life.

Ms. Z: I see what you're saying. I could feel a surge in my guilt with a feeling of needing to protect him. And I do miss him, too. I'll wait a bit before I decide to rush down there. I'm supposed to go down there on Friday, and I'll see how it's going.

In this instance, the therapist suggested that Ms. Z aid her daughter by promoting Valerie's mentalization of her son, a way of furthering the use of these skills.

Mentalization Skills in Challenging Low Self-Esteem

An additional use of mentalization is considering positive experiences and responses from others, particularly for a patient who has an intensely negative self-view. Some patients have such severe self-critical feelings that they can reject, deny, or shut out knowledge of others' positive views, even though it would ease their distress to take them in. Patients can use their mentalization skills to consider these positive views and how they contrast with their own self-criticism.

CASE EXAMPLE: MR. AA'S INTENSE SELF-CRITICISM

Mr. AA, a 62-year-old White salesclerk, who suffered from chronic depression, was highly self-critical about his capacity to function effectively at his job and in his relationship with his wife and son. However, he was able to maintain his work in sales, and with his wife's job as a social worker, they were able to manage financially. In addition, he had a fairly good relationship with his son, although he worried that he would be a poor role model for him. Mr. AA's negative self-view emerged in his early home life, in which his mother was critical of his capabilities and his father had little to do with him, focusing instead on his own work and hobbies. Mr. AA's self-criticism was so severe that it emerged quickly in the transference, worrying that he would be "fired" by the therapist for an anticipated "failure" in therapy. To challenge these self and other representations, the therapist explored discrepancies in his self-view from what occurred in his life and how others saw him. The following exchange happened in the fourth session of PrFPP:

THERAPIST: You have said that you think of yourself as a failure and incompetent, but I'm puzzled about your view given your financial contribution to the family and your relationship with your wife and son.

MR. AA: I think you might be assuming something too positive. My wife makes most of the money.

THERAPIST: I understand that, but I'm not sure how that makes you a "failure." Additionally, I'd like to hear more about your relationship with your wife, which from what you said so far, is positive.

MR. AA: It's overall pretty good. I think I depend on her too much, and she gets annoyed about it at times. But she depends on me for child care, which she does appreciate.

THERAPIST: That's very curious given your intense self-criticism. Many people who come to my office have major problems in their marriages and with their partners, whereas yours is actually going fairly well. What does she think of your view of yourself as a failure?

MR. AA: She gets tired of hearing about it. I mean, she doesn't think it really makes sense. These days, I don't mention it much because it annoys her.

THERAPIST: How would you describe your relationship with your son?

MR. AA: As you know, 8-year-old boys often look up to their father, so it's fairly positive. I try to hold back on my negativity when I'm around him. It sometimes slips out.

THERAPIST: I don't think every 8-year-old boy admires his father. I think you might try to keep in mind more what your wife and son think about you. Because you've so powerfully internalized your mother's intense criticism and your father's lack of interest, you're not able to think of yourself other than negatively. We need to build a place in your mind where you can step back from this negativity. We can certainly start with their much more positive view of you.

MR. AA: I can try to keep that more in mind, but the way I feel is so strong that I tend to dismiss any positives. I just keep thinking that I'm going to fail.

By working with his mentalization skills, the therapist helped Mr. AA consider positive views of himself in an effort to reevaluate his self-loathing and his expectation of rejection. Indeed, the fact that he had been married to his wife for many years, without major disruptions, further demonstrated how his negative expectations were overstated. This formulation formed a basis for addressing his depressive symptoms and self-loathing.

CASE EXAMPLE: MR. O'S SELF-LOATHING

Another example of use of mentalization to modulate a propensity to feel devalued or self-critical occurred with Mr. O, the patient whose judgmental, harsh father died suddenly when he was 12 (see Chapter 4). The patient struggled with feeling better off with his father's death, which caused significant guilt. Subsequently, Mr. O viewed himself as a failure in accord with his father's very high expectations of professional success, despite having done quite well in his jobs. At the same time that he saw himself as a failure, he would become furious when he felt others devalued his work. Indeed, these experiences caused interpersonal conflicts at work that eventually led to his being fired.

Having lost a job recently led to a worsening of his depression, with even more intense feelings of failure. The therapist interpreted how he accepted his father's excessive and problematic standards (only professional success mattered) while at the same time despising his father's values. Additionally, his rage at his father, which created guilt, would become self-directed. However, he had a resurgence of anger at feeling devalued when he was offered a new job from a colleague developing his own business at a salary that did not meet his expectations.

MR. O: I don't really even see the point of taking this job at that salary.

THERAPIST: Well, you've said you needed the money, and we know you're more negative about yourself when you're unemployed. Maybe this indecisiveness has to do with your anger at feeling devalued.

MR. O: I am furious about that. It's below what's usually paid for that position. What do they think I am? A garbage collector? I've had some very high-level jobs.

THERAPIST: Despite which you describe yourself as a failure. But we know that, when you feel your skills are devalued, you become very hurt and angry. We've discussed how you have to be careful about how you express your feelings about this with others.

MR. O: Oh, yeah. Now I'm terrified about what I'll say. But so far, I've handled things okay. I talked to him about how I felt, but he said that's all he could do for now. But why doesn't he just say he doesn't care about me?

THERAPIST: I think that's taking the offer very personally. And that maybe it feels like your father rejecting you. But I wonder if the salary offer has something to do with the business being one that he's starting up. Do you know how the business is doing or what his financial situation is?

MR. O: I don't think it's turning much of a profit yet. It's a start-up.

THERAPIST: I wonder if you could consider the possibility that it's the status of his business, or his own financial situation, that's leading him to offer that salary. Not that he intends to devalue you. Just the fact that he wants to hire you under these conditions indicates he respects your work and feels you can contribute.

MR. O: Then he has a weird way of showing it. I'll consider what you said. I hadn't thought of it that way. But I'm pretty angry about it.

Mr. O cycled between intense feelings of failure and inadequacy and a grandiose view of his capabilities and what he could expect from others (Kohut, 1971). Due to failures of mirroring by his parents, he was not able to develop realistic expectations of himself and his capabilities. This led to an alternation between severe feelings of inadequacy and feeling enraged about being devalued. Working to obtain a broader sense of what might be going on with his colleague in offering the salary he did was in part an effort to empathize with him and help mentalize another perspective that could enable him to step back from this cycle.

CASE EXAMPLE: MR. BB'S BLACK-AND-WHITE THINKING

Mr. BB, a 32-year-old Asian tech worker, struggled with depression and obsessive-compulsive disorder. The therapist pointed out the pattern of black-and-white thinking he had with regard to his evaluation of himself and others, viewing people as either successes or significant failures. He tended to see himself as a failure, despite having a tech job at a major company, as his standard of success was someone who "runs a hedge fund." The therapist pointed out the extremes in his thinking, and Mr. BB was able to reconsider how he made this assessment. Similarly, he would describe women as either highly intelligent and attractive or as someone he wasn't interested in. This led to significant problems in his dating, particularly as he felt that a highly attractive woman would not be interested in him, and his high standard ruled out many women he might pursue a relationship with.

In exploring these all-or-none standards, the patient recalled a girlfriend he had had for over 3 years whom he described as attractive and with whom he developed a good relationship. The therapist worked with this information to point out that his all-or-none standard was not always present and not the most helpful for developing relationships. The therapist explored what Mr. BB liked about this woman:

MR. BB: She was nice, and she really cared about me. She was interesting, too.

THERAPIST: What was the reason you broke up with her?

MR. BB: Actually, she was a Jewish girl, and in my family, my mom has made it clear that we need to marry someone who is Catholic.

THERAPIST: You feel that you have to follow that standard?

MR. BB: My mom is kind of pushy about it, but she has a good point. You're going to share more with someone of the same religion.

THERAPIST: It's hard to tell if that's more your idea or something you feel from family pressure.

MR. BB: I hadn't considered that so much.

In the next session, the patient came in expressing a realization about his mother:

MR. BB: You know, when we had that discussion about the pressure to marry someone Catholic, I thought about it. I realized that my mom pressures me in a lot of ways that maybe have more of an effect on me than I thought. She's always asking if a girl

I'm dating is attractive, or Catholic, and she's been kind of pushy about my career. She encourages me to push for a promotion or maybe look for a better job at another firm. I kind of like the job I have.

THERAPIST: That does seem to be related to your all-or-none feeling. Do you have any thoughts about what motivates her viewpoints?

Here, the therapist is encouraging the patient to use his mentalization capacities to consider why his mother put this pressure on him. An alternative approach would be to have the patient consider why he feels the need to accept his mother's standards.

MR. BB: That's a good question. Thinking about it, she's kind of competitive with other people. She engages in one-upmanship. Like she's better than other people. If someone says they're sick, rather than being empathic, she says, "I know someone else with that disease." And people in my neighborhood brag about their kids. Maybe that's why she's pushing me about this. People say my kid has this or that job. Or maybe she wants me to be seen with a pretty girl.

THERAPIST: That's interesting because it seems like she's really intending for you to do the best you can, maybe based on her own standards and motives. It certainly sounds like this contributes to your view of yourself, women, and jobs as either failures or successes. Your old girlfriend and your job don't fit these poles, although you feel positively about both of them.

MR. BB: One thing I liked about Rachel was that I felt she accepted who I was. She thought my job was fine. And she didn't give me any trouble about my OCD symptoms, like my family often does. I felt like she just cared about me.

THERAPIST: So, this may be important in terms of what you're looking for in a relationship: someone who accepts who you are and doesn't pressure you about their expectations.

In this case, the therapist encouraged the patient's mentalization skills, which led him to an understanding that his mother pressured him with her own expectations. These pressures contributed to the patient's polarization of failure and success, adding greatly to his anxious and depressive symptoms. These interventions helped the patient begin to reconsider his expectations of himself and others, reducing his sense of pressure and dissatisfaction. For example:

MR. BB: You know I've thought more about my old girlfriend, and there were a lot of good things about the relationship. She wasn't the most attractive person around, but I found her attractive. And she cared about me. She never really expressed any negative judgments about me. This really contrasted with my mom. I didn't realize the pressure I felt from her. I need to reconsider who I decide to date.

And on the occupational front:

MR. BB: Actually, I have a pretty good job. It's not running a hedge fund, but it's interesting. And I don't need to work all the time, like some people do. I like having free time to follow my own interests.

Using Mentalization to Address Relationship Problems

Mentalization skills can be invaluable in addressing relationship problems, as they aid the individual in understanding the other person's perspective.

CASE EXAMPLE: MS. CC'S EXPECTATIONS OF REJECTION IN RELATIONSHIPS

Ms. CC was a 46-year-old single White social worker with a long history of struggles in relationships with men. She would recurrently become involved with charming, highly articulate, successful men who ultimately turned out to be very self-focused. Recurrently, she would end up feeling rejected and unappreciated by them. The therapist and she identified that these men bore similarities to her father, a highly successful doctor, who at times was intensely engaged with the patient, alternating with a disregarding or contemptuous attitude toward her. The therapist interpreted that these relationships were a form of repetition compulsion, in which the patient hoped to develop a relationship in which she symbolically conquered her father's narcissism and gained his interest. Thus, it became clear to Ms. CC that she needed to look for a partner different from her father who was better able to have a give-and-take relationship.

Ultimately, she became interested in Ted, a lawyer who was intelligent and caring but did not have the charm of the other men she had been attracted to. Although initially she found this unappealing, she stayed with the relationship, as she realized the problems that men with more charming characteristics had caused for her. As she dated him, she became increasingly attached, believing that she had found the man with whom she could have a long-term commitment. However, she began to feel that Ted did not adequately express his positive feelings toward her. She missed the intense expressions of warm regard other men had displayed, downplaying its inconsistency. Indeed, she took his lack of positive expression as disregarding and rejecting of her. In discussing Ted's history, she reported that he had grown up in a nearly affectionless home, with little positive feeling. This lack of affection had occurred after the death of his brother from an accident, which deeply impacted him but that the family rarely spoke about.

The therapist explored if she had addressed this issue with Ted. Ms. CC said she had not, as she was quite convinced his behavior showed that he did not care. However, the therapist encouraged her to discuss his behavior with him to get a sense of his response.

Thus, Ms. CC told Ted she was upset about his not having followed up after she had gone to the doctor to discuss a possible breast biopsy.

Ms. CC: I told him I was very hurt that he didn't call me after the doctor's visit, and I felt it showed that he didn't care. But he was actually shocked that I felt this way. He said he deeply cared about me and just assumed I would call him if there was a problem.

THERAPIST: How did you feel about his response?

Ms. CC: Very relieved. I mean he came across as really caring. Doesn't it sound like it to you?

THERAPIST: It does. But we should also try to understand why you're not convinced and need reassurance from me.

Despite this relief, her hurt and anger returned, and she felt recurrently disappointed in his level of engagement with her. For instance, he continued to be less solicitous than she hoped and rarely expressed his love toward her. The therapist worked on mentalization skills with Ms. CC to assess whether her reactions made sense with regard to Ted's behavior.

THERAPIST: I wonder if Ted is just not capable of thinking proactively to take these steps. You described him growing up in a cold household. Maybe he defends himself from expressing such feelings.

Ms. CC: I hadn't really thought of that. You're suggesting that he feels that way, but he just can't remember to express it?

THERAPIST: Yes, because it would help explain how, when you confront him regarding this issue, he does express it. And I think we need to consider how vulnerable you feel about this. If you're not reassured, then you tend to assume that you're being rejected based on your father's behavior toward you.

Ms. CC: I see what you're saying. But isn't that still a problem if I need this kind of response, and he can't do it?

THERAPIST: Yes, it is, but it's not necessarily the same problem you thought you had: that he's not rejecting you, just having trouble expressing his feelings in a way that reassures you.

Here, the therapist combines developmental interpretations with an emphasis on mentalization to help the patient understand the intensity of her reaction and her potential misperception regarding Ted. The patient had further talks with and observations of Ted that provided her with more evidence of how he struggled to be in touch with his feelings based on his own traumatic background.

Using Mentalization in Addressing Marital Conflict

CASE EXAMPLE: MR. DD'S ESCALATING FIGHTS WITH HIS WIFE

Mr. DD, a 48-year-old White business executive, had recurrent conflicts with his wife in which he reported criticisms from her that he felt were unfair and over the top. He would typically respond by attacking her, leading to fights that would disrupt their relationship for days.

MR. DD: I didn't clean the counters, and my wife just went crazy on me! She was screaming, "How could you not do that?" Then she said I didn't love her and that I never loved her. Can you believe that? Equating not cleaning counters with not loving her? That's so way over the top!

THERAPIST: She certainly sounds very critical of you and catastrophic about the relationship. How did you handle it?

MR. DD: Not very well. I called her a crazy bitch. Then of course she got even more furious. She said, "See what I mean?" I ended up sleeping on the sofa, and we haven't talked since then.

THERAPIST: I certainly hear how you get furious toward her and the cycle escalates. Perhaps it would be helpful for me to talk with your couples counselor to understand these issues better.

MR. DD: I think that's a good idea.

In addition to his psychotherapy, Mr. DD had entered into couples counseling with his wife. Through these treatments, Mr. DD gained a better sense of why his wife got so angry. In addition, by having a conversation with the couples counselor, his therapist gained a better sense of the problems in the marriage. The couples counselor confirmed the patient's view that his wife would suddenly and unfairly attack him, but the patient would typically retaliate. The couples counselor worked to disrupt what she called "the negative cycle." One of the approaches to doing this was to explore the wife's background, which was highly traumatic. The patient had mentioned some of the wife's experiences but did not know the full extent of her traumatic history. Part of the couples and individual therapy was teaching the patient mentalization skills to better understand his wife's attacks, which stemmed in part from these traumatic experiences.

MR. DD: I guess I'm coming to understand better just how traumatized my wife was. I didn't realize the intensity of the fights between her parents, and the physical and verbal abuse toward her. Her father left when she was 8, which was in many ways a good thing. But then her mother had to go to work and left her to care for her two younger siblings. I think this was really too much for her. I guess that's why she says she expects more of me, but she always ends up disappointed.

Developing Mentalization Skills 147

THERAPIST: It sounds like in some ways she expects you to compensate for what she experienced, which of course you can't fully do. But I think this helps us understand why she becomes so furious at you when you forget to do certain chores because she had to manage too many chores growing up.

MR. DD: I hadn't thought about it that way. But I can't always do what she says. As far as she's concerned, I should be running around the house all day doing chores.

THERAPIST: It sounds like your wife perceives you as if she's back in the traumatic state. She sees you as behaving like her neglectful and abusive parents, leaving her feeling overwhelmed. Perhaps it would be good to address this in couples counseling.

MR. DD: That makes a lot of sense. Understanding these things about her has helped me be less intense in my attacks, and the fights have been shorter. I think understanding that she's reacting as if she's in the traumatic state might help both of us to calm down.

EXPANDING THE USE OF MENTALIZATION SKILLS

As patients learn mentalization skills, the therapist hopes that they will begin to apply them independently to new situations. Ongoing practice using the worksheet can help patients consider new opportunities to use mentalization.

CASE EXAMPLE: MS. R'S DEMANDING BOSS

Ms. R, discussed in Chapter 5, demonstrated how she was putting into use her mentalization skills. She was chronically troubled by her boss's intense pressure, demands, and criticism regarding her technical work. As far as Ms. R was concerned, her work was an area in which she had been successful and helped compensate for areas of her life in which she felt inadequate. She felt disdain for her boss, whom she saw as a typical manager who had little understanding of her technical work and could not properly assess her accomplishments. She would express criticism toward him, sometimes leading to interpersonal struggles. At the same time, even though she disrespected his views, she would experience a surge of insecurities about this area of her life that she could normally count on. Finally, she would feel guilty about the intensity of her anger and the struggles that ensued.

On working with mentalization approaches, however, Ms. R was able to consider what her boss might be dealing with:

MS. R: I realized the other day what kind of pressures he must be under. The company's pushing to get this project done and putting the heat on him. He's really dependent on me, as he doesn't quite understand the technical aspects of what needs to be done, yet he's under tremendous pressure to have these tasks completed. He could get fired if they're not done by the deadline!

THERAPIST: So, how has this affected your perception of him?

MS. R: I think he may be putting the heat on me because of this pressure. He's probably mad at his bosses and taking it out on me.

THERAPIST: Well, that's a thoughtful perspective. How does this affect your experience of the critical things he says?

MS. R: I feel kind of bad for him. I mean it's not okay to be taking it out on me, but if I don't get things done, he gets in trouble. I think it's helped me be less angry with him. And it's helped keep in mind how capable I am. I can do the work, but if the company's expectations are unreasonable, what am I supposed to do?

THERAPIST: That's a good approach, and you seem quite a bit calmer about it.

MS. R: And I still recognize he's a jerk, but I've stepped back a bit from fighting with him. I've said, "Look, this is what we can do."

Ms. R's increasing mentalization skills helped her in dealing with her boss and also aided in improving her self-esteem, as she better understood her boss's critiques as coming from his own insecurity, rather than her incapacity to perform a task. The several cases presented in this chapter show how patients can be taught mentalization skills, increasing their capacity to observe themselves and others, and how these skills can be used to manage and relieve a variety of problems.

In the next chapter, I describe building a formulation for problems based on emotions and contexts, developmental history, self and other representations, conflicts and defenses, and mentalization deficits and how to use this formulation to address problems.

QUESTIONS AND IDEAS TO THINK ABOUT

1. Consider the patients you are working with and whether these patients use mentalization skills. Do you notice an impact on their relationships with others? On their mental health in general?

2. With a patient that you are working with who is feeling attacked or rejected by someone, have the patient consider what might be going on with the other person. What are the results of this exercise? Was it helpful to the patient?

WORKSHEET 6.1

Understanding What Is Happening in Your Own and Others' Minds

These questions will help you and your therapist identify and understand what is happening in your own and others' minds. Skills in considering this information will be used to better address your problems.

What are the problems you have with one of your relationships and your feelings about it?

Consider the feelings and problems you are having from the other person's perspective. What responses can you imagine the other person might have?

How do you understand the differences in perspective you have with the other person regarding the problem in the relationship?

(continued)

From *Skills Training in Psychodynamic Psychotherapy*, by Fredric N. Busch. Copyright © 2026 The Guilford Press. Permission to photocopy this worksheet, or to download and print additional copies (www.guilford.com/busch-forms), is granted to purchasers of this book for personal use or use with clients; see copyright page for details.

What Is Happening in Your Own and Others' Minds *(page 2 of 2)*

If someone is criticizing or judging you, what do you think might lead that person to react the way they do? Pick a specific instance or two to consider.

When that person criticized you, how much did it have to do with you, and what might be going on with the other person?

In a recent conflict you had with someone, what do you think that person might have been reacting to?

CHAPTER 7

Clarifying the Psychodynamic Formulation and Using It as a Framework of Interventions

This chapter describes how to organize information about dynamic factors that contribute to problems, described in the prior chapters, into an overarching psychodynamic formulation (Perry et al., 1987). Therapists and patients work to identify these factors, including the context, emotions, and functions of problems, self and other representations, developmental history, internal conflicts and defenses, and mentalization difficulties. The formulation is also used to determine how different and overlapping aspects of these dynamics contribute to various problems. Understanding these interconnections, where present, can aid the patient and therapist in relieving these difficulties.

Additionally, this chapter demonstrates how to use the formulation as a framework for targeting problems. Thus, therapists choose interventions based on the formulation and use them to modify the psychodynamic factors that contribute to problems. In addition to communicating aspects of the formulation verbally, the formulation can be written in the form of a worksheet (see Worksheet 7.1: Identifying Contributors to Your Problems, pp. 170–171; all worksheets are available at www.guilford.com/busch-forms) that spells out a problem list, dynamic contributors, and interventions that possibly can be shared with patients.

In considering whether to share a written formulation directly with the patient, such an intervention may be particularly useful for patients who have difficulty recognizing and "taking in" clarifications and interpretations of their dynamics. It may also be helpful for patients struggling to understand links between their problems and dynamic factors. Such difficulties can be caused in part by defensive efforts in patients who avoid acknowledging painful inner states or memories. A written formulation gives additional opportunities to overcome these defenses.

The formulation is developed and changes over the course of therapy to include new understandings of and interventions for the patient's problems and their dynamics. A second worksheet (*Worksheet 7.2: Assessing the Impact of Treatment*, pp. 172–173) can be used to spell out the patient's understanding and recognition of their problems, how they have addressed contributors, and changes that they have made. Case examples are used to demonstrate the elaboration of the formulation and its use as a framework for interventions.

CASE EXAMPLE 1: MS. EE'S FEELINGS OF INADEQUACY AND INCOMPETENCE

Ms. EE was a 62-year-old White divorced financial advisor with a history of recurrent anxiety and depression. These episodes would be accompanied by a sense of incompetence, with a fear that she would be unable to accomplish even quotidian tasks, such as shopping for groceries, creating intense anxiety. In addition, she was highly self-critical that she was having these difficulties, accusing herself of being childlike and needy in her struggles ("It's wrong for an adult woman to be having these kinds of problems"). These episodes would often be triggered by a visit to her mother and siblings. Her mother typically placed multiple demands on the patient, asking her to take care of several chores in the house and accompany her to doctors' appointments. Although Ms. EE recognized her mother's aging and need for help, she noted that her mother had always made such demands and easily could have obtained help from others in doing these chores. She was particularly frustrated and hurt when her mother reacted disdainfully to the patient's revealing her anxiety and depression, and her need to take breaks from chores, as her mother told her to "buck up."

In addition to these anxious and depressive symptoms, Ms. EE suffered distress from bullying by her younger brother and sister. They would often criticize her for not doing more to help their mother, even though their mother expected little of them, and would sometimes exclude Ms. EE from family events. In this way, they sided with the mother's criticism of the patient. Furthermore, Ms. EE tended to become overly responsible with friends, to her own detriment. For example, she would spend significant time and energy taking care of them when they were ill. She would often end up feeling taken advantage of and demoralized by the time and efforts these tasks required.

Exploring the Contexts and Emotions Surrounding Problems

In the case of Ms. EE, the therapist noted that contextual triggers involved intensive efforts to help her family members and her friends struggling with problems, which set off pressures to yield her own needs to those of others. In exploring her recent resurgence in symptoms, the patient reported that they began when she took her younger brother for surgery and spent time caring for him in his recovery. The therapist and patient noted the link to pressures she felt when she was young to care for others (see the next section, Developmental History). When she focused her energy on caretaking, she developed feelings of incompetence and fears that she would be unable to handle issues in her daily life, displaced from her childhood fears of being unable to manage her responsibilities. She also took care of her brother despite his treatment of her. The therapist interpreted that her anger at him became directed toward herself in her self-criticism.

Developmental History

Ms. EE reported that her mother was often ill and in bed when she was growing up. The patient believed, retrospectively, that her mother suffered from depressive episodes. She expected Ms. EE to assume the primary care of her younger siblings by the time she was an early adolescent. The patient recalled feeling terribly frightened about being able to manage the younger children, particularly the youngest, a 4-year-old. Any attempt, however, to obtain more help from her mother was met by her mother's rage, yelling that she would just have to find some way to manage. Ms. EE would end up feeling guilty about even trying to get her mother to care for her. Bullying by her younger siblings also began as she entered adolescence and was tolerated by her mother. Her father, often at work, remained disengaged from her mother's behavior.

Self and Other Representations

The therapist and patient identified three core problematic self and other representations: the self as needy with others being judgmental; the self as needing to care for others with others as demanding; and the self as insecure with others powerful and bullying. The therapist linked the patient's self and other representations to her developmental history, in which she accepted her mother's demands and viewed her inability to meet these expectations as related to her own inadequacy. This insecurity and guilt led her to tolerate punishment in the form of her mother's criticisms and her siblings' bullying. Notably, the patient's academic skills and subsequent work led to her being admired by her father and other family members, as professional success was highly prized in the family.

Conflicts and Defenses

Ms. EE struggled with anger at her mother, which triggered intense guilt, and would result in her denying these feelings, directing them toward herself in self-loathing for being too "needy." In addition, she would suppress the anger she felt and become overly caring for others, a form of reaction formation. Furthermore, she would deny or disparage her own dependent longings, which were a source of intense conflict.

Mentalization Impairments

Ms. EE's mentalization skills were disrupted by her expectations of criticism by others and her own intense self-attacks. Thus, she had difficulty considering why her mother and siblings behaved the way they would toward her. Contributing factors to their harsh attitudes included her mother's dependency on the patient and her siblings' competitiveness with her academic achievements.

Below is the formulation of her problem list, as well as contributory dynamic factors and interventions (described in the case history below) as identified by the therapist and patient over the course of several sessions. *(For this listing of problems, dynamic formulation, and interventions, you may find it convenient to use Worksheet 7.1: Identifying Contributors to Your Problems, pp. 170–171)*

Problem list: What difficulties has your treatment focused on?
1. Anxious preoccupation with feelings of incompetence
2. Intense guilt and self-criticism
3. Bullying by siblings
4. Overresponsibility

Triggering contexts and feelings: What situations and feelings trigger or exacerbate these problems?

Feeling anxious during visits with her family, pressured to take care of friends in need of help.

Developmental history: What types of experiences in your past may have had an influence on these problems?

Mother was often ill and in bed, expecting patient to take care of younger siblings when she did not feel capable. Father was disengaged.

Self and other representations: How do you understand yourself, and how do you understand others insofar as they've had a bearing on these problems?

Self as needy; others as harsh, judgmental

Self as needing to care for others; others as needy, demanding

Self as insecure; others as powerful, bullying

Conflicts and defenses: What feelings and wishes have you struggled with, and how have you attempted to manage them?

Conflicts

Anger at others for their demands become turned against the self, viewing herself as not responsible, inadequate. Guilt about needing help from others.

Defenses

Denial of her own anger, projection onto others, viewing them as critical of her.

Reaction formation in her care for others toward whom she is angry. Denial of her own needs.

Mentalization impairments: Do you consider how others are thinking when they behave in ways that are upsetting to you?

Due to self-blame, she has an inability to recognize how siblings' bullying may stem from jealousy or how her mother manipulated her into feeling she should do all the work.

Interventions based on the formulation: What have you and your therapist discussed about how to manage your problems?

Identify triggers as relating to demands of family or others needing help, understanding what happens internally (feeling pressured) in response to these triggers.

Recognize how the patient is now able to manage chores, that she is not incompetent, as opposed to childhood.

Identify harsh self-criticism patient feels toward herself for "neediness," as related to internalization of her mother's attitudes. Present alternative positive views of her attitudes and behavior.

Link pressures of overresponsibility she feels with family and friends as related to her mother's demands, expectations, lack of empathy.

Identify inability to recognize and confront bullying as based on her own internalization of expecting punishment for feeling "inadequate." Address the threats she believed would occur if she confronted bullying.

Psychotherapeutic Interventions Using the Formulation

As aspects of the psychodynamic formulation are identified, the therapist uses these as a framework targeting contributors to problems. Thus, the therapist addresses the contexts and feelings surrounding problems, developmental factors, relevant self and other representations, contributing conflicts and defenses, and mentalization impairments. The description that follows demonstrates how these factors were addressed in the case of Ms. EE.

Addressing the Context and Feelings Surrounding Symptoms

The therapist suggested that the current precipitating circumstances of her symptoms triggered painful experiences from when Ms. EE was growing up. The therapist linked the intense and out of proportion fears of being incompetent in managing day-to-day expectations to traumatic situations in which she felt overwhelmed by pressures to care for her siblings. In contrast to her fears, he pointed out that she was in a different position now and quite capable of handling her daily chores.

Addressing Self and Other Representations

Ms. EE would often insist that she was a "bad person" deserving of other's negative judgment, including the therapist's. The therapist presented positive alternative views, referencing her work success and devotion to her friends, and noted that the level of harshness with which she treated herself was not rationally based. The therapist worked on how to avert the onset of the whirlpool of self-negativity, including managing the level and type of contact she had with her family and the negative self-views it triggered.

Addressing Conflicts and Defenses

The therapist interpreted that another component of her self-loathing was generated by her conflicted anger toward her mother, which became directed toward herself. Furthermore, Ms. EE felt like a bad person for having any wishes for support from others. Indeed, she nearly cried when a doctor she was seeing expressed concern about her welfare, as noted in the following vignette. The therapist linked these conflicts to her early environment where any expression of anger or longing for care was responded with harsh criticism and punishment.

MS. EE: And I couldn't even decide whether to take a bus or my car to see the doctor. It's a simple decision, but I was all worried about it. And I started crying when the doctor was supportive of me. Now you have to admit that's really messed up.

THERAPIST: It's easy to see why you would cry because, given your history, you would be affected by someone trying to help you. But you're very self-critical about the difficulties you were having.

MS. EE: Well, come on. For a woman my age to be that anxious and needy. That's messed up.

THERAPIST: My sense is that you can't tolerate your wishes for help because you became convinced growing up that they were bad. You had to accept your mother's viewpoint because otherwise there was no way to get along with her. In fact, she would attack you for complaining about having to care for your siblings and make you feel terrible.

MS. EE: I do think I'm bad. And I don't really think I had a tough childhood, not compared to many kids in the world. They don't even get their basic needs met!

THERAPIST: Again, you're minimizing your struggles, as if psychological factors can't have a severe negative impact. It's just difficult for you to wish to be taken care of without feeling terribly guilty.

MS. EE: I see what you're saying. And I would like to take a break. Maybe a massage would be a good thing. But then I feel I don't deserve it!

THERAPIST: We have to continue to help you accept that having needs and receiving support is not a bad thing!

MS. EE: Okay, I'll try the massage. Let's see what happens.

Addressing Mentalization Impairments

In working to improve her mentalization skills, the therapist addressed the problem of her acceptance of her siblings bullying:

THERAPIST: Why do you think they bully you?

MS. EE: Because I deserve it, I think. They know from my mom that I'm kind of a screwup.

THERAPIST: But how could you be a "screwup" if you're so successful with your work and friends?

MS. EE: I guess that doesn't count.

THERAPIST: I wonder if you ever considered the possibility that they're jealous of your success?

MS. EE: No, I hadn't thought about that. Why would they be jealous?

THERAPIST: Your success is a focus of admiration by other members of your family, and it was by your father. Maybe you allow their bullying in some way as a punishment.

MS. EE: I've never thought of it as allowing their bullying, but I can see how you might see it that way. But the jealousy idea makes more sense to me. They could be mad because I'm admired by the family for my professional work.

The dialogue above shows a shift in the formulation of Ms. EE's problems as the experience of bullying as something that happened that she could not stop to something she unconsciously allowed based on her sibling's jealousy and a feeling that she should be punished. This shift ultimately led to Ms. EE no longer tolerating or accepting this bullying.

Use of the Transference

In the transference, Ms. EE felt as if the therapist was criticizing her and viewed her as a bad and irresponsible person, mirroring her own view. The therapist responded that he did not see her as "bad" in any way, although she felt an undue degree of responsibility, based on her guilty feelings. In her traumatized state, she would react disdainfully to the therapist's reassurance, responding "You can't be serious," and present more examples of her "badness." However, as she began to build more of a zone of safety and with the therapist's persistent nonjudgmental and encouraging stance, she began to incorporate more positive self-views and expectations from the therapist.

CASE EXAMPLE 2: MR. FF'S FEAR OF CONFRONTATION

Mr. FF was a 52-year-old gay White engineer with a history of recurrent anxiety and depression. He reported that his recent bout of symptoms began when he and his husband Albert were planning to buy a new house. They had been renting a house in which the patient was quite comfortable, but his husband had wanted to purchase a house for investment purposes. He had a resurgence of depressed and anxious mood and became preoccupied when he realized that, for financial reasons, the new house would be smaller than their current apartment. He believed he would feel confined, as they lived with their two children, a daughter in high school and a son who was living at home after graduating from college. Mr. FF felt angry at Albert for what he perceived as pressuring him to move but reported that he was particularly threatened by confrontation and would avoid it if at all possible. He spent increasing time alone in his bedroom or in the kitchen cooking and listening to music on his headphones. His husband had described him as "resentful," and Mr. FF acknowledged that he probably was.

Exploring the Contexts and Emotions Surrounding Problems

Mr. FF had a resurgence of anxiety and depression in the context of the purchase and planned move to a new house. He felt angry and anxious about the changes that would occur, including a reduction in space, but did not feel safe addressing them with his husband for fear of damaging their relationship.

Developmental History

Mr. FF, in exploring his background, described his father, a hardworking lawyer, as being tough and domineering with the patient. His father was irritable with intermittent rages in which he accused his children (the patient, his brother, and his sister) of being lazy or "bums." The patient described feeling very angry at his father but was fearful of confronting him, even as an adult. For instance, Mr. FF did not defend his daughter when his father started to become judgmental toward her, commenting on her weight and clothing. His mother was caring but entirely yielding to his father.

Self and Other Representations

Mr. FF viewed himself as weak and needing to submit to others who were more powerful on the one hand and feared damaging others with his anger on the other.

Conflicts and Defenses

Mr. FF feared that any expression of his angry feelings would damage others, and therefore he avoided confrontation. This fear partly stemmed from his identification with his father, whose anger he experienced as deeply hurtful. He ended up expressing his own anger passive-aggressively, isolating himself from others and appearing sullen.

Mentalization Impairments

Mr. FF could not consider that others could be responsive to his needs, as he anticipated attack or rejection.

From the dynamic factors identified in the exploration of symptoms and the patient's developmental history, the therapist identified these components of the psychodynamic formulation:

Problem list
1. Depressive symptoms
2. Anxious preoccupations
3. Passive-aggressive withdrawal
4. Tensions with husband

Triggering contexts and feelings
Frustration and anxiety about moving to a smaller house and his son living at home.

Developmental history
Tough, domineering father with intermittent rages. Accusations of children being lazy and irresponsible. Angry at but highly fearful of confronting father.

Self and other representations
Self as weak; others as critical, judgmental
Self as aggressive; others as easily damaged

Conflicts and defenses
Conflicts
Anger as intolerable and frightening, anticipating he would damage others.

Defenses
He linked his own anger with his father's (identification with the aggressor), fearing his anger would be damaging like his father's or lead to damage or rejection. His anger was expressed passive-aggressively.

Mentalization impairments
His intense fears of retaliation interfered with him considering that his husband would want to address his concerns about the house.

Interventions based on the formulation
Identify patient's frustration with current family situation and planned move.
Recognize how patient withdraws in a passive-aggressive way rather than address his frustration.
Link patient's fear of and guilt about expressing his frustration to his developmental history
Identify that patient overestimates the risks of addressing his frustrations.

Addressing the Context and Feelings Surrounding Problems

Recognizing the move and frustrations with his husband as triggers, the therapist explored whether Mr. FF had addressed his concerns about the house with Albert:

THERAPIST: Have you talked with Albert about your concerns?

MR. FF: No, I haven't. I mean, I don't want to get him upset. He's wanted this house for a long time. And I don't like confrontation.

THERAPIST: What troubles you about the house?

MR. FF: First, I don't want to move. I'm completely comfortable in our current house, which is large and spacious. I'm doing this for him. And my kids want to do this, too. But I don't think any of them are considering that the house will be smaller and how we'll be more crowded together in it.

THERAPIST: Are there other things frustrating you?

MR. FF: Yes, but I can't think of any examples.

THERAPIST: Let's see what comes to mind.

MR. FF: We got a new dog. I didn't really want the dog that much, but they did. And this past Saturday my kids and husband went to a ball game. The dog got sick, and I had to take it to the vet. I was looking forward to time on my own and didn't get to do anything I wanted. I guess I was thinking of more freedom as I got older, and now I just have more responsibilities.

THERAPIST: You do sound very frustrated about this. Any other issues?

MR. FF: I just don't want to be around my husband and kids that much.

THERAPIST: Can you say more about why?

MR. FF: Not really. I'm not really getting anywhere today.

The therapist was surprised at Mr. FF's comment given that he was providing valuable information, and Mr. FF appeared very uncomfortable. The therapist also believed Mr. FF's hesitation represented the transference, in that Mr. FF feared confronting him.

THERAPIST: I'm surprised to hear you say that. I'm certainly getting a better idea of what's troubling you. I wonder if it's because you feel uncomfortable talking about how angry you are, even with me.

MR. FF: Yes, I feel guilty about being so angry. I feel bad that my son's home from college and I don't want to be around him. First, he always sides with my husband, and he thinks he's right about everything. And I don't want to be taking care of him, but his friends moved away, so he needs a lot of support. Obviously, I can't tell him how I feel.

THERAPIST: That's a lot of things frustrating you about him. It seems like you're feeling trapped. You have these pressures and demands, and you can't really express them because you feel guilty. Also, you've said you don't want to have any confrontations. So, you retreat to your bedroom and the kitchen.

MR. FF: Yes, I do feel trapped. And it will be even worse in the new house. What am I supposed to do about it? How do I get better at communicating this to them?

THERAPIST: I think it's important to understand why you feel so guilty and fearful about being angry. This would help to identify why you feel so threatened about addressing your concerns.

MR. FF: I guess that could have to do with my father. I was never allowed to confront him.

Addressing Developmental Factors/Self and Other Representations/ Conflicts and Defenses/Mentalization Skills

In the following sequence, the therapist linked Mr. FF's self and other representations, conflicts and defenses, and mentalization impairments to his history and considered how Mr. FF might address his feelings with Albert.

THERAPIST: It makes sense that your fears stem from your father's rages and harsh judgments, but these circumstances are different now. It feels important to address your concerns and frustrations about the house, even though you're frightened about doing it. Otherwise, you just get more anxious and depressed.

MR. FF: Yes, but I don't want to hurt Albert or end up being retaliated against.

THERAPIST: I understand that. But I wonder if you're overly concerned about that. Maybe because of the harsh way your father expressed criticism toward you. It's hard for you to consider that addressing frustrations with someone could be helpful rather than damaging.

MR. FF: Maybe. I'm pretty mad right now. I could try to address the issues with Albert and see how it goes. But just as I'm about to do it, I tend to balk.

THERAPIST: You should consider making notes about what happens at that point. You can use the diary (see Worksheet 3.1: Monitoring Circumstances, Thoughts, Feelings, and Reactions Surrounding Problems, p. 76) to keep track. Then we can figure out how to address the threats you experience when you feel so angry and trapped.

Using this information, Mr. FF addressed his concerns about the new house with his husband and the pressure he felt to move forward with the plan. Although he was highly anxious when he first started talking with Albert, the discussion did not create the feared interpersonal conflict Mr. FF expected. Albert was responsive to his anxieties regarding space and discussed how they might stop the plan. However, after raising his concerns, Mr. FF became much less angry about the move and was able to better recognize the positives of the plan. He subsequently reported liking the house after they made the move. As the therapist shifted to address problems with his son, Mr. FF felt safer than previously describing his frustrations with him.

CASE EXAMPLE: MR. F'S WORKAHOLISM

Mr. F, described in Chapter 2, was an accountant who was anxious due to his excessive workload. However, he felt unable to turn down new clients to reduce the pressure he felt. In addition to his anxiety, he struggled with conflicts with his wife, particularly regarding his unavailability. Finally, he had a tendency to drink excessively. The details of his history were described in Chapters 2 and 4. After 16 sessions, the therapist devised the following formulation using Worksheet 7.1: Identifying Contributors to Your Problems (pp. 170–171):

Problem list
1. Compulsive working
2. Generalized anxiety
3. Conflicts with wife
4. Alcohol use

Triggering contexts and feelings

Problems worsened by the pressure he felt to accept new clients and his increasing workload.

Developmental history

The patient reported his father as having been demanding and irritable, often complaining that the patient was irresponsible and demeaning the patient's social and intellectual capabilities. In middle school, Mr. F rebelled via use of pot and avoiding studying, although he anticipated his father would punish him for these behaviors. He developed strong feelings of social anxiety and inadequacy. However, he ultimately shifted his attitude toward school and improved his academic performance, getting into an excellent college, followed by being hired by a high-level accounting firm.

Self and other representations

Self as inadequate; others as demanding

Self as angry, rebelling; others as duped or punitive

Conflicts and defenses
Conflicts

Anger as potentially damaging; directed inward.

Psychodynamic Formulation as an Intervention Framework 163

Defenses

Denial of anger at others, which became self-directed. Anger projected onto others, viewing others as critical, punitive. Denial of work pressure, minimizing impact on his life.

Mentalization impairments

Mentalization disrupted by Mr. F's intense achievement pressures, leading him to deny his own conflicts and pressures and minimize his wife's frustrations.

Interventions based on the formulation

Identify anxiety triggers as linked to pressures to achieve, overwork, and conflicts with his wife.

Identify how the patient minimizes the adverse impact of demands he placed on himself, including by using alcohol to ease his stress.

Have patient make efforts to decrease work to identify and manage factors that impelled him to overwork.

Understand the impact of his father's attitudes as related to self-imposed demands for overwork and wishes for approval.

Address feelings of inadequacy with countering evidence of the patient's effectiveness and successes, addressing the question of why these feelings persist.

Explore inability to feel angry at father despite excessive demands placed on him and minimization of his efforts. Recognize how his anger becomes directed toward himself, internalizing his father's negative views of him.

Help patient to understand his wife's anger in relation to the pressures he placed on himself.

Addressing the Context and Feelings Surrounding Problems

One of the interventions, discussed in Chapter 3, focused on efforts to reduce his workload and using these attempts to identify and better manage contributory factors. This approach was based on a notion that the patient compulsively accepted additional clients, even when overworked, to suppress or relieve certain feelings and fantasies. The approach, using Worksheet 3.3: Exploring Not Acting on an Impulsive Behavior (pp. 78–79), was described for Mr. F's case in Chapter 3. As Mr. F increased his efforts to turn down work, he struggled with intense emerging emotions and fantasies that identified additional contributors to his problems and aspects of the psychodynamic formulation.

Mr. F's feelings included a fear that somehow his business would fall apart entirely if he rejected a single client, although he acknowledged this did not make rational sense. A second component was anxiety anticipating that he would feel empty or bored during the day when he was not working with clients. Third, he felt a responsibility for clients as soon as they requested his help. He stated that many sought him out because they had trouble with their prior accountants and needed his help to manage difficult situations. He felt guilty about turning them down because he felt unsure that they could otherwise get the help they needed. Finally, he believed that turning down work would lead him to "fall short" of his father's expectations of accomplishment, lowering his self-esteem. However, he found that when he did reject clients, he primarily felt relieved rather than anxious or down. The therapist addressed how he was increasingly confronting these fears in the following exchange:

THERAPIST: So, with regard to your excessive workload, you mentioned you've been taking some of the steps we discussed to try to address it.

MR. F: For one thing, I've really shifted in how I think about it based on my better understanding of what a problem it is for me and observing what I've been experiencing. I've started to think about how to avoid taking on new clients rather than just automatically accepting them. When I begin to feel the pressure, worrying about losing business, I try to remind myself how busy I am. When I worry that I won't feel as good about myself if I'm less busy, I remind myself how relieved I actually feel. I work to confront these fears rather than just accept them.

THERAPIST: It sounds like your perspective has really shifted and you have a framework from which to address the problem. So, you've recognized at first being busy boosts your self-esteem, even though it subsequently drops?

MR. F: I do feel it makes me important somehow. And you know growing up I felt inadequate. I mean, not very popular, not one of the smart kids, and girls rejected me. Now I do feel more successful. In fact, I think Susan likes flirting with me in part because she thinks I'm a big shot. But then I lose that "important" feeling when I start struggling to keep up with my work.

THERAPIST: Sometimes people feel inadequate from a lack of interest or involvement from their parents, and we know that your father either wasn't very focused on you or was very judgmental. But what he did admire was people who worked very hard and made a lot of money.

MR. F: And what did I do? Rebelled by not working hard in school! But now that I'm more successful, I try to keep that in mind and confront my feelings of inadequacy.

THERAPIST: How do you think he'd feel about your work now?

MR. F: I wish he were around to see it. I think in a way he'd admire it, but I'm not sure that he would feel it's enough. I mean, to be a success in his book took some pretty intense efforts.

THERAPIST: So, maybe that's what helps you to feel better for a little while: being even busier and adding new clients helps you feel recognized for your skills. So, you could finally feel admired by your father. But then it just gets to be too much, and instead of feeling positive, you feel anxious, inadequate, and pressured.

MR. F: I can see more now how it's connected to him and that I create stress for myself in some way to please him. But it's kind of sad if I were pressing ahead with all this effort, and having these conflicts with my wife, just to impress him. I ended up feeling worse. I feel better when I can get my work done.

Addressing Self and Other Representations, Conflicts, and Defenses

The transference became valuable for these purposes when the patient began to fear the therapist would judge or punish him for his difficulty making progress turning down referrals. When the therapist responded in an empathic rather than critical manner, recognizing how difficult these struggles must be, this material could be further used to confront his negative self and other representations. It subsequently emerged that Mr. F was angry at the therapist for what he viewed as pressuring him to change his behavior. The therapist accepted his feelings and interpreted how, due to conflicts about his anger, he ended up directing it toward himself as unfair criticisms about his difficulty cutting down his workload.

Addressing Mentalization Impairments

As noted, Mr. F's capacity to think about how others reacted to him was disrupted by his pressure to achieve and overwork. With regard to his marital problems the therapist addressed the use of mentalization in an effort to improve Mr. F's skills and better respond to his wife's frustrations.

THERAPIST: In considering the tensions with your wife, what do you think about her anger at you?

MR. F: It's really frustrating that she doesn't recognize that I need to stay late at the office sometimes. She benefits from the money I make and then gives me a lot of trouble.

THERAPIST: But I guess from what we've learned she has a point. You are working harder than you need to. And she gets frustrated by your absences.

MR. F: Yes, but it still feels critical. I see what you're saying. It's my being preoccupied with work and coming home late that she gets mad about.

THERAPIST: We've learned that you also get angry about all the work you have to do. But then you take it out on her, even though you're now in basic agreement with her, as you've acknowledged that you're driven to overwork.

MR. F: You mean at this point we're really in agreement. I hadn't thought about how we're both bothered by the same thing. Maybe I should talk to her about it.

THERAPIST: I think that would be a good idea. That may help relieve the tension.

Addressing Interconnectons between Problems

As noted previously, different problems often share dynamic contributors or one problem could develop in an attempt to manage another. In the formulation developed for Mr. F, the contributors to his various problems were found to be interconnected. For example, his feelings of inadequacy and pressures to achieve led to overwork, drinking, and the flirtation with his administrator. His overwork created tensions with his wife, and his anger at his work became displaced toward her. His generalized anxiety stemmed from both the pressure to overwork and fears he would get into trouble for being distracted or not completing his tasks. Furthermore, his alcohol use represented an effort to manage his anxiety, while ultimately exacerbating the pressure and the conflicts with his wife. Understanding these interconnections aided in developing strategies to address Mr. F's various problems. For example, reducing his work pressure helped to ease his irritability and better manage his drinking. Interventions that address core dynamics contributing to various problems can often have a ripple effect in relieving these difficulties.

REPETITION COMPULSION IN RELATION TO PAST ADVERSE OR TRAUMATIC EVENTS

Individuals may sometimes unconsciously recreate events related to past trauma or adverse experiences (Freud, 1920). This phenomenon, known as repetition compulsion, can function as a way for individuals to manage situations in which they felt helpless or out of control. They unconsciously attempt to obtain a better outcome from the traumatic experience by exerting control over situations in which they previously felt helpless but can create recurrent problems or possible retraumatization in doing so.

For example, therapist and patient identified a pattern in which Mr. F accepted so much work that he struggled to do what was essential. At some point on most days, he had a wave of fear that he would be unable to complete the tasks he needed to do. He would become preoccupied with intrusive thoughts about how clients would be angry at him for not getting their work done. However, by the end of the day, he would find some way to finish the job, providing intense feelings of relief. Thus, he would put himself at risk of getting into "trouble," anticipating punishment, followed by feeling rescued and that he behaved like a "good boy."

In this way, he recreated painful experiences with his father in which he would suddenly be reprimanded for being "irresponsible." However, these reprimands were capricious, and it was not clear which tasks he had not fulfilled. Thus, when his father was in an irritable mood, he lived in fear of being suddenly punished without reason, although he ended up accepting the view of himself as "irresponsible." Thus, in his day-to-day behaviors, he recreated this fear, which he felt helpless to manage as a child, but gained control over it by somehow getting enough done to be able to please his clients.

THERAPIST: So, what's your understanding of this behavior?

MR. F: I thought it was just work I needed to do, but I realize now that I kind of create these situations by taking on more work than I can comfortably manage. When it's going well, it's kind of exciting. But when it's too much, as it often feels like, I start to get panicky and wonder how I'll get it done. Then I feel the relief of completing it.

THERAPIST: It sounds almost like a drug effect.

MR. F: I guess so. And then I drink at night to relieve the stress. Also, I'm worried I'll get depressed and bored if I can easily complete the work. There's something exciting and scary about doing it this way.

THERAPIST: So, it's interesting that you recreate the conditions of anxiety you felt growing up, but in these circumstances, you have more control over it. You end up relieved and avoid punishment. You put yourself at risk of being viewed as irresponsible and then avoid that accusation.

MR. F: I didn't realize I might somehow be repeating these struggles from growing up. It does get very dicey. Maybe all this fear isn't necessary. I know my efforts to cut back clients have provided some relief from these anxious episodes.

ASSESSING THE IMPACT OF PrFPP

In addition to observing the impact of PrFPP in psychotherapy sessions, the therapist may want to make a more formal effort to determine what the patient has understood about his problems and the impact of this knowledge. In addition, such efforts help patients to make a similar determination and can aid them in formalizing their understanding. The approach outlined here can be used to evaluate the impact of therapy on the patient's understanding of their problems and related dynamics. (See Worksheet 7.2: Assessing the Impact of Treatment, pp. 172–173, for a convenient tool for doing this assessment.) The information you glean from this assessment can be used to help determine which problems are improved or only partially resolved and need to be addressed further. Such an evaluation can also help determine whether patients have improved enough to consider terminating treatment (see Chapter 9). Examples are provided of Mr. F's responses to these questions.

> **What are the problems you've identified with your therapist that you are working on in therapy?**
>
> I've understood better what a problem my overworking has been for me. I know it's made me anxious, but I didn't recognize the level of pressure it creates for me. I just rationalized it as necessary.

How has your thinking about these problems changed with therapy?

Now I get how overwork has affected various aspects of my life, upsetting my wife and leading me to drink to try to manage the stress. I also realize that I'm driven to do this. I thought it was something I wanted to do.

What have you understood about contributors to these problems?

I understand now that my history with my father continues to affect me. I didn't recognize the level to which I was still trying to impress him, how this would drive me, even though I lost him years ago. I thought it was just money and success, but it's like I'm carrying this around with me, along with the pressure to achieve to get his approval.

Are there particular situations that tend to trigger or exacerbate your problems?

Definitely. The greatest stress is when I'm not sure I can get the work done that I need to. I'm worried my clients are going to be mad at me for not completing the tasks they need done. I also get anxious when potential new clients call me on the phone. I know now it's not a good idea for me to take them on, but I've had a terrible time just saying no. It's almost like I feel I'm responsible for them.

Have you recognized aspects of your history that contribute to your problems?

I get that this need to please my father drives my overwork. I hadn't made that connection before. The only people he really admired accomplished a lot. Otherwise, he was always accusing you of being lazy and irresponsible.

Do you have a sense of how you view yourself and your expectations of others in relation to the problems you have and how that's changed?

I've ended up putting myself under pressure to please others, trying to get done what they need done. I guess I always feel on the verge of disappointing others, and I need to push myself to overcome it. It's like I'm going to be punished, and I just avoid it by pushing myself more.

Do you recognize internal struggles (conflicts) that contribute to these problems?

I've understood that I end up directing my anger at my father toward myself. It's like I'm blaming myself for what I haven't done instead of appreciating what I have accomplished. I guess I never felt safe recognizing how angry I am about what he did to me. And I've put my wife in a position of punishing me by getting her mad at me for being too busy.

What are the ways you've learned that you defend against these struggles? Do these defenses contribute to or relieve your problems?

I realize I try to defend against stress by drinking to calm my nerves, but that just makes things worse. Also, flirting helps distract me and makes me feel better. But then I feel guilty about it.

In what ways have you found that your ability to think about what's happening in your own or other's minds affects the problems you have?

I've blamed my wife for not getting it, being mean to me. Or not recognizing what I've achieved. But now I understand that her concerns have been on target. She has some of the same worries that I have. I'm less mad at her, and she realizes I empathize with her more. We've been doing better, and my flirtation has cooled off a bit.

This chapter has demonstrated the value and use of a psychodynamic formulation that identifies contributors to problems, and the use of the formulation as a framework with which to identify interventions. The problem list, formulation, and interventions shift and change over the course of treatment as additional information emerges about patients and initial approaches have an impact. Thus, PrFPP identifies and targets a range of contributing factors that enable a broad set of interventions to ease problems and reduce vulnerability to recurrence.

Having developed and used interventions to address dynamic factors that contribute to problems, the next focus is on further reducing patients' problems in the working-through process. Approaches to diminishing patients' vulnerabilities to recurrence of problems are described. A worksheet to identify further targets for addressing problems is discussed.

QUESTIONS AND IDEAS TO THINK ABOUT

1. With a patient you are working with, try devising a psychodynamic formulation with a problem list, contexts and feelings surrounding problems, developmental factors, self and other representations, conflicts and defenses, and mentalization impairments. Is this formulation helpful to your thinking about the patient? If so, in what ways?

2. Using the formulation you made in Question 1, devise a series of interventions based on this formulation. Had you considered these interventions before?

WORKSHEET 7.1
Identifying Contributors to Your Problems

These questions will help you and your therapist formulate—that is, recognize and address—links between your problems and factors leading to them.

What difficulties has your treatment focused on?

What situations and feelings trigger or exacerbate these problems?

What types of experiences in your past may have had an influence on these problems?

(continued)

From *Skills Training in Psychodynamic Psychotherapy*, by Fredric N. Busch. Copyright © 2026 The Guilford Press. Permission to photocopy this worksheet, or to download and print additional copies (www.guilford.com/busch-forms), is granted to purchasers of this book for personal use or use with clients; see copyright page for details.

Identifying Contributors to Your Problems *(page 2 of 2)*

How do you understand yourself, and how do you understand others insofar as they've had a bearing on these problems?

What feelings and wishes have you struggled with, and how have you attempted to manage them?

Do you consider how others are thinking when they behave in ways that are upsetting to you?

What have you and your therapist discussed about how to manage your problems?

WORKSHEET 7.2

Assessing the Impact of Treatment

These questions will help you and your therapist determine which problems are improved or only partially resolved and need to be addressed further. In addition, they provide information about understandings you have gained about your problems.

What are the problems you've identified with your therapist that you are working on in therapy?

How has your thinking about these problems changed with therapy?

What have you understood about contributors to these problems?

Have you recognized aspects of your history that contribute to your problems?

(continued)

From *Skills Training in Psychodynamic Psychotherapy*, by Fredric N. Busch. Copyright © 2026 The Guilford Press. Permission to photocopy this worksheet, or to download and print additional copies (www.guilford.com/busch-forms), is granted to purchasers of this book for personal use or use with clients; see copyright page for details.

Assessing the Impact of Treatment *(page 2 of 2)*

Have you recognized aspects of your history that contribute to your problems?

Do you have a sense of how you view yourself and your expectations of others in relation to the problems you have and how that's changed?

Do you recognize internal struggles (conflicts) that contribute to these problems?

What are the ways you've learned that you defend against these struggles? Do these defenses contribute to or relieve your problems?

In what ways have you found that your ability to think about what's happening in your own or other's minds affects the problems you have?

CHAPTER 8

Working Through

Working through (Freud, 1914) in psychodynamic psychotherapy or psychoanalysis is a gradual process in which patients gain increased understanding of their dynamics along with a growing recognition of how these factors affect their symptoms and problems. This phase is important in reducing problems as well as vulnerability to their recurrence, as an expanding psychodynamic formulation and interventions are used to address contributing factors. In the psychoanalytic situation, the process includes the therapist giving interpretations of similar dynamics as they apply to different manifestations of problems and various circumstances in which they occur.

Working through happens outside of therapeutic sessions as well, as patients consider what has been understood in treatment and recognize how it applies to their lives. For instance, for patients with severe anxiety disorders, who frequently perceive themselves as disempowered or helpless, part of working through involves a recognition of their fearful dependency and the threat anger or assertiveness presents for them. As the threat from their anger diminishes, they feel increasingly safe asserting themselves, enabling others to respond better to their needs. For example, in the case of Ms. S below, the patient's recognition of panic being triggered in situations in which she felt stuck and helpless enabled her to recognize the frustration caused by being a club chairperson and taking steps to alleviate this situation.

In PrFPP, working through focuses on building aspects of the psychodynamic formulation that contribute to problems and addressing these factors. Thus, the therapist and patient consider the following components in developing further information and interventions: contextual and emotional triggers, developmental history, self and other representations, conflicts and defenses, mentalization impairments, and behavioral problems. Goals include having an additional impact on symptoms as well as behavior and relationship difficulties and developing skills to address problems and reduce the risk of recurrence. Worksheets identifying these parameters and interventions can be of value, along with assessments as to what changes patients are making. *The approach described in this chapter, which is called Elements of Working Through Problems (see Worksheet 8.1, pp. 190–191, as well as other worksheets, online at www.guilford.com/busch-forms), can be used for the therapist and patient to evaluate the progress they are making in working through problems. Sample responses to the worksheet are provided in some of the cases below.*

CASE EXAMPLE: MS. S'S RESURGENCE OF PANIC

Ms. S, described previously in Chapter 5, reported a resurgence of panic with a trapped feeling during a movie she attended. In exploring the context surrounding this panic episode, she described the film as including intense angry fights in the context of family conflicts. Through previous exploration, she recognized this anxiety as being linked to her father's temperamental behavior, which triggered her view that anger was dangerous, leaving her feeling frightened and helpless. She also experienced a surge of worry that someone in the play was going to have a heart attack. When she associated to these fears, she recalled her grandfather's heart attack and death from cardiac complications when she was 8 years old. Her panic fear often focused on something being wrong with her heart, but she had not previously linked this to her grandfather. Further exploration revealed her belief that anger was a significant contributor to heart attacks, something she had read about in the newspaper. Indeed, she recalled that her grandfather suffered from high blood pressure and had temperamental outbursts, not unlike her father.

This increased understanding of the relationship between angry feelings and expressions and heart attacks helped to ease this episode of panic and her fear that something was wrong with her heart. At this point, she associated further to the trapped feelings of her panic attacks and her father's angry outbursts, in which she felt threatened by his demands. She began to identify anxiety in situations in which she felt pressured, helpless, and angry, including with difficult bosses at work. She recognized, for example, that she was experiencing these feelings in a club where she was a member. She was head of a committee that would arrange speakers for the club. However, whenever she made suggestions, there was typically someone or a group of people who objected, based on either lack of interest or the political views of the speaker. If she pushed forward with the speaker, she felt that some of those who objected continued to hold it against her or became cool socially. She recognized that she found being the chairperson a thankless task, reminiscent of the situations that caused panic with difficult bosses at work. Having identified the role as likely to trigger panic, she questioned why she remained in it. She made a determination that she should resign from the chair and the committee.

Ms. S: So, I told them I was resigning, and of course they asked me to stay on. And like the good girl I usually am, I told them I would think about it. Then I was thinking if they really need me, maybe I should stay on.

THERAPIST: So, what did you decide?

MS. S: I began to get a surge of anxiety about remaining in the role. Then I remembered what we discussed. How you said I didn't have to yield in situations where I felt frustrated or stuck in. So, I wrote back and told them that I thought they needed to get a new person in the role. I felt so relieved afterwards. Looking back, I didn't realize how angry I was.

THERAPIST: Can you describe what you were angry about?

MS. S: Definitely. At all the people who complained. I was just trying to do my job and get interesting people to speak, and they objected for all these petty reasons. I feel infuriated even thinking about it now. I must have suppressed it before.

THERAPIST: It seems like you're feeling safer with your angry feelings and that helped you more readily recognize the problems at the club. You recognized that situations in which you feel helpless and criticized aren't good for you or your anxiety. You may have felt it was necessary for you to do them just as you felt pressured to respond, as you did to your father's angry demands.

MS. S: It hadn't occurred to me before that I could find a way out.

Below are the therapist's notes from his exchange with Ms. S, for which he relied on guiding questions from Worksheet 8.1 (pp. 190–191), describing factors involved in her working-through process:

Further information about triggers of problems: Ms. S recognized that her being chair at the club was one of the situations that was a trigger for her anxiety and panic. She came to realize that she was not as helpless as she believed in these situations, and she was able to make changes, such as resigning from the position.

Increased understanding of developmental history and its impact on current perceptions and problems: She increasingly recognized that situations in which she felt helpless were related to her experience growing up with her temperamental, judgmental father, in which she was helpless but needed to be differentiated from current circumstances in which she was not.

Ongoing addressing/confronting problematic self and other representations: She further confronted her view of herself as helpless, with others as controlling and judgmental, recognizing that she was not as helpless and others were not as critical as she thought, or that she did not always have to accept their judgment.

Further addressing areas of conflict, problematic defenses: She continued to address her conflicts surrounding anger, including the belief that anger was dangerous, harmful, and disruptive to relationships. These conflicts had led to denial and suppression of her anger. She learned that recognizing her anger and finding a more effective way to express it helped to reduce her panic symptoms.

Identifying mentalization impairments and building mentalization skills: Her expectations that others would be judgmental and critical limited the flexibility of her mentalization. Addressing these impairments helped her to consider that others might be acting out of jealousy or fear when they behaved in judgmental and controlling ways.

Ongoing use of the transference: Ms. S perceived the therapist as benign and caring, supporting her not feeling trapped and effectively expressing her frustration, in contrast to representations of her father as harsh and judgmental.

Shifts in behavior—assertiveness: She made increased efforts to assert herself in panicogenic situations, those in which she felt helpless and unfairly put upon.

Ongoing development of skills to address problems: Learning to self-observe feelings of powerlessness, along with greater safety with her anger, helped her to identify situations in which she felt helpless and criticized and act on this recognition.

CASE EXAMPLE: MS. GG'S BURDENS

Ms. GG, a 68-year-old White divorced woman with two children, presented with depressive symptoms in the context of feeling overburdened by work in the family business. She reported initially enjoying her retirement from a public relations firm 10 years previously with travel and time spent with friends. However, a relative who was running the family business, from which Ms. GG received funds, became too impaired to manage it. Although others were part of the enterprise, she took over the bulk of the responsibilities. Unfortunately, the business involved much more work than she anticipated, and she quickly realized that it had been poorly managed. She began an effort to correct the significant problems that had developed in accounting, costs, and repairs of various facilities involved in the business. She found herself spending long hours completing these tasks and began to withdraw from social activities in order to do so. She increasingly felt lonely, frustrated, and down.

At first, she simply accepted that it was her responsibility to take on these tasks, but when she started to consider getting help, she felt guilty about asking others to contribute. This included her two children, as she did not want to disrupt their involvement in their careers and marriages. Given the heavy workload, she realized the best solution was to sell the business. However, when she attempted to proceed with the sale, other family members blocked it, as they were not willing to accept the offered price, which was lower than they expected.

The therapist noted a pattern of accepting too much responsibility, feeling guilty about trying to off-load some of the work, and then feeling depressed and trapped. As they explored her history, developmental factors emerged that contributed to her over-responsibility, particularly being pressured to care for her mother, who struggled with debilitating cancer treatments when she was an adolescent. Her father made it clear that it was her job to take on this role, reprimanding her for any attempt to "buck" her responsibilities. She remembered getting furious with her father but then feeling guilty about causing difficulty when her parents were struggling. Ultimately, the patient dealt with her anger toward her parents by suppressing it and directing it toward herself, blaming herself and her younger brother for her mother's struggles. She felt that perhaps her mother would have been less exhausted if she did not have children to take care of.

In further exploring her conflicts about anger, Ms. GG reported a surge in self-criticism after she lost her temper with her friend Jennifer. She was organizing a birthday party for another friend at her house. Jennifer approached her and asked to give a speech that included comments about an incident Ms. GG believed the friend might find embarrassing. She responded firmly: "I wish you wouldn't," and the friend walked away without much comment. Afterwards, Ms. GG was highly self-critical and ashamed that she had "lost her temper" and called Jennifer to apologize. Although Jennifer appreciated the apology, she went on to criticize the way the patient had arranged the speakers at the party. Rather than being angry, Ms. GG blamed herself for the criticism because she had "attacked" Jennifer initially.

Ms. GG: I thought you might believe I was too self-critical about how I responded to Jennifer.

THERAPIST: Do you think that may be the case?

Ms. GG: Possibly. But I lost my temper, and I was verbally violent. I didn't explain to her why I said what I did, so I think I'm to blame here.

THERAPIST: Calling it "verbally violent" seems kind of harsh. Look, you were trying to manage the party at your house, and Jennifer suggested an idea you truly believed would be embarrassing. People do get mad sometimes.

Ms. GG: It helps me to have that perspective, but it's hard for me to see it that way. But then I know I get very down on myself about things many people wouldn't think twice about.

THERAPIST: We've discussed how you struggled with your anger toward your parents when you had to care for your mother. It does appear as if the guilt about these difficult circumstances growing up has had a broader effect on you.

Ms. GG: That may be. I didn't realize how guilty I tend to get, even when it's understandable that I'd get mad!

THERAPIST: We are working on building a place in your mind to which you can step back and consider that you might be getting too self-critical. I think it shows how unacceptable you find it to get angry, and this leaves you struggling to assert your needs with others.

Ms. GG: I think that makes sense. But I can tell you another situation where I made progress with my brother, letting him know how I felt about a decision regarding the business. And I didn't get mean!

THERAPIST: That shows you're using your understanding of your anger to address problems more effectively.

As she came to feel safer about her anger toward her parents and recognized factors from her childhood that led her to overassume responsibility, she began to shift in her attitude about selling the business. She told others family members that it would need to be sold, as she was unable to handle her current tasks, and it was creating problems with her mental health. Although some family members were frustrated with this plan, they ultimately agreed because they also did not want to manage the business. The therapist and patient determined that it was important to watch out for this tendency to take on chores in other settings that were not required of her. With this perspective in mind, she turned down planning a retirement party for a former colleague, stating, "Someone else can take care of it." She experienced feelings of relief and liberation in discharging these tasks.

CASE EXAMPLE: MS. J'S SHOPPING COMPULSION

Despite progress in her therapy and a reduction in her impulsive shopping, Ms. J continued to spend more money than she earned. In the working-through process, the therapist made further efforts to link her buying sprees to feelings of being deprived and angry at others. One source of these feelings was fights she had with her husband, who criticized Ms. J for "nearly putting us in the poor house," and "being a spendthrift."

MS. J: I just get furious with him. He doesn't get that I make my own money, and I can spend it how I want to. And he's a real downer. He just walks around the house moping.

THERAPIST: Well, does he have a point? Are you able to afford the things you're buying? I know you said you've struggled to get out of debt.

MS. J: Yes, there's concerns, but I don't like the way he says it, calling me names. It actually makes me want to shop more rather than less.

THERAPIST: It sounds like you feel angry and deprived by him and want to rebel, which we know are just the feelings that tend to trigger your shopping. But it sounds like he may have reason to worry about your financial situation. Maybe he has trouble handling his own feelings about it.

MS. J: It's kind of annoying to hear you say that. But I hadn't thought of it that way. And then I think, "He's not going to set limits with me. I'm just going to shop anyway."

THERAPIST: We should talk about your feeling angry with me because maybe you're seeing me as depriving. And we've talked about how angry and deprived you felt about your mother abandoning the family. But we want to help you better manage these impulses.

Ms. J: I guess I have to learn to get a hold of these feelings. They get me into trouble. And I know he's not like my mom. He's stayed with me despite my problems.

In this exchange, the therapist further linked her perceptions and frustrations with her mother to those with her husband, helping her to see the differences between them. This technique involved another way to bring her developmental history to bear on the present and confront her representations of her husband as similarly depriving.

Below are aspects of the psychodynamic formulation and interventions the therapist used to target her feelings and shopping impulses:

Further information about triggers of problems: Ms. J continued to learn more about situations that caused her to feel angry and deprived, including the reactions of her husband. She used this awareness to better manage her shopping urges.

Increased understanding of developmental history and its impact on current perceptions and problems: Ms. J gained further understanding of how her experiences with her mother led her to perceive her husband as more depriving and less caring than he actually was.

Ongoing addressing/confronting problematic self and other representations: She gained further understanding and ability to address her perceptions of herself as deprived and others as withholding and uncaring. The therapist presented an alternative view of her husband as worried but ultimately supportive of her, easing the tensions in their relationship and helping to manage her feelings of anger and deprivation with him.

Further addressing areas of conflict, problematic defenses: Ms. J increasingly recognized the lack of safety that she felt in needing things from others to avoid the hurt and pain she experienced from her mother's rejection. As she felt safer with these wishes, she became more able to directly communicate her needs with her husband.

Identifying mentalization impairments and building mentalization skills: The patient had difficulties considering her husband's source of distress, instead simply viewing him as depriving. This tendency involved her proneness to perceive others as depriving and her anger overriding her having empathy for his anxiety. The therapist made increasing efforts to improve her mentalization and recognize her husband's legitimate financial concerns.

Ongoing use of the transference: Ms. J became able to recognize that she would tend to experience the therapist's efforts to help her stop spending as an attempt to deprive her rather than help her to manage her impulses.

Shifts in behavior: impulse control: Ms. J's increased understanding of her pressure to shop helped her hold off on acting on these impulses.

Ongoing development of skills to address problems: Ms. J's use of Worksheet 8.2 helped her develop alternative strategies for managing her feelings of deprivation and anger.

In further working through efforts aimed at behavioral change, the therapist suggested that she withhold the impulse to go shopping for at least 30 minutes after she experienced it. Rather than simply being a behavioral intervention, the therapist suggested that she observe and write down her experiences and feelings during that time. The goal of this exercise was twofold: to understand better the pressure she felt to go shopping and to further build the capacity and a framework to hold off on impulses to buy things. During this exercise, she described feelings of anxiety, dysphoria, and deprivation, along with strong impulses to stop the exercise and go shopping. (Worksheet 8.2: Holding Back on Impulsive Behaviors, p. 192, is useful for doing this exercise.)

The therapist worked with her to consider how she might better tolerate these feelings. One approach was to consider the link to her mother's depriving behavior, but the patient did not find this to help relieve these urges. Better interventions for her included exercise, which aided in reducing bodily and mental tension, and contacting a friend to speak to. Talking with a friend also helped to relieve her emotional deprivation, particularly her friend Olivia, who also had a traumatic background and struggled with drinking urges. The patient found her to be particularly valuable in empathizing with her struggles.

WORKING THROUGH MR. A'S PRESSURE TO RESPOND TO THE NEEDS OF OTHERS

As noted in prior chapters, Mr. A's panic attacks occurred in the context of feelings of aloneness and isolation as well as feeling pressured by others. One aspect of working through included continuing to develop his awareness of these triggers. He increasingly recognized when he felt that others were being controlling and intrusive. These situations included his husband's and son's intrusive advice and friends' and colleagues' preoccupation with certain topics or activities that they expected him to respond to. At these times, he recognized an experience of bodily tension and mounting anxiety associated with the pressure, along with a wish to remove himself.

Dealing with these situations and the associated panic attacks involved further shifts in representation of self and others. The link between pressure he felt from others and demands to hear his father's "lectures" and his father's temper episodes became increasingly clear. He challenged the self-view that he had to submit to others' pressures. This opened up the space for him to challenge others' expectations or at least have a conversation. He felt relieved when making decisions or communicating to others that he wanted space to be on his own, when he could "be himself."

As the therapist had him associate further to the tension in his body, they recognized that these states included both anxious and angry feelings. In these situations, he was both anxious that he had to respond to others and angry that they were expecting him to do so. The belief that it would be damaging to others to let them know that he did not want to do what they wanted him to do related to fears that his anger would cause damage. The patient's conception of anger included it either being expressed in a hurtful or temperamental way, like his father, or being submerged, as he did with his father and others. The increasing sense that anger could be expressed in a safer manner in negotiating his needs enabled him to more effectively address the intrusiveness he experienced with his husband and son and pressures from others to yield to their topics or activities.

Increasing mentalization skills helped him to consider why others were pressuring him. For instance, he identified that his son had his own anxieties about how to express certain feelings, making him overly wary about the patient's behavior. Thus, Mr. A was able to discuss such concerns with him and encourage his son to seek therapeutic help.

In the transference, he became fearful when he had to cancel a series of sessions to complete his own projects. He had the fantasy that the therapist would criticize him for taking too much time away from therapy, in part based on the therapist's own needs. He described a prior therapist who pressured him not to cancel sessions, stating that "I thought he had more of a problem than I did." Thus, they could explore how his feelings and fantasies regarding asserting his own wishes emerged with the therapist. He felt increasingly safe expressing his need to attend to his own work when necessary and less fearful of the therapist's judgment and anger. Increasingly, he felt safe communicating such needs to others, including with humor. For example, he told a friend who demanded that he listen to a long story, "Boy, you're really stuck on this, aren't you? I actually have to go now."

WORKING THROUGH IN PrFPP: MR. A

Further information about triggers of problems: He increasingly identified feeling trapped by others' needs and preoccupations, including his son's and husband's worries about him taking proper care of himself, making comments about how he should live his life.

Ongoing addressing/confronting problematic self and other representations: The therapist challenged his view of himself as needing to submit to demanding, needy others.

Further addressing areas of conflict, problematic defenses: Therapist and patient addressed fears that anger about feeling pressured would hurt others, push them away or cause rejection, triggering panic.

Identifying mentalization impairments and building mentalization skills: Frustration and anxiety made it difficult to consider why others pressured him. He recognized that his son had his own anxieties about what was safe to express to others.

Ongoing use of the transference: Mr. A was fearful that the therapist would react negatively to canceling sessions to pursue his projects. They confronted his fear that the therapist would pressure him to come based on his own needs.

Shifts in behavior: assertiveness: He felt increasingly able to assert his own wishes and express his needs without fear of hurting others.

Ongoing development of skills to address problems: Increased recognition of angry feelings in response to pressures from others enabled him to challenge his fear of his anger and assert himself more.

MR. M'S REASSESSMENT OF SELF-WORTH

Mr. M, discussed in Chapters 3 and 4, viewed himself as "bad" whenever he had trouble with his business or thought he was not making enough money. These circumstances would plunge him into a severe depressive, anxious state. These negative feelings and self-perceptions were identified as deriving from his development, during which he believed his parents viewed him as "bad" except for his precocious business skills. One line of intervention in the working-through process involved reassessing how he determined the value of himself and others. Rather than being based on the business achievements alone, he increasingly recognized the importance of helping and supporting others. He realized that he did not want others to experience the lack of caring and responsiveness that he did. Thus, he made more efforts to support others in his environment emotionally and financially. The significant impact he made in helping others, including family and employees, provided another tool for the therapist to confront his self-view as bad.

When he talked about his efforts to support others, he would typically become tearful. Exploring these feelings led to identification of two sources of his tears: one in which he was affected emotionally by seeing the relief of others' distress and the other which represented mourning the loss of what he did not get. This mourning process helped to further clarify the lack of emotional support from his parents and its impact on him. This understanding helped to ease the pressure he felt to succeed in business in an intrapsychic attempt to gain his parents' love.

As he reconsidered his conceptions of what made a person worthy, he began to reassess his attitudes toward his children, which included being disappointed in their business skills. Relations between them were fraught as he would make judgmental comments about their jobs and how they ran their lives. However, as his representations of self and others shifted, he began to understand their areas of struggle in their lives rather than judge them. He shifted toward a more supportive and collaborative relationship with them, working to help them deal with their problems rather than criticize them. These efforts began a steady shift in a positive direction as their trust in him increased, further promoting his positive self-view.

As his relationships became more collaborative, he worried such an attitude would lead him to be "weak" rather than "tough" in his business dealings, as his impact partly stemmed from others being fearful of him. However, he came to recognize that he could be tough when necessary, without being mean or bullying. These steps further aided his self-esteem, as bullying others would sometimes lead to a backlash in which he felt guilty about being too "scary." Indeed, he began to recognize that he could spend time strategizing about what his client would be influenced by and use that information to reach his goal. This shift involved increasing his mentalization skills, considering what was going on in the mind of the person he was dealing with. He found that sometimes being friendly or complimentary to those he negotiated with was more effective than consistently using a "tough" posture.

Working further on the impact of his developmental history and intrapsychic conflicts, he increasingly became aware of the intensity of his anger at his parents. He had minimized these angry feelings as he directed them toward himself, accepting the view of himself as "bad" rather than focusing on the problems with them. Gaining a better awareness of his anger helped him to manage temper outbursts he had toward others whom he experienced as ignoring him, realizing it reproduced the injury he felt with his parents. At the same time, his mentalization skills helped him gain a fuller picture of his parents' difficulties, stating, "They weren't ready for a kid like me." Awareness of his anger also helped him to mourn his disappointment with his parents and realize that he could now receive the appreciation and recognition he could not as a child.

However, he continued to worry at times that his business would have inadequate profits and at certain points, particularly when money that was due to him did not come in, he had a significant drop in mood. The therapist worked with him using the whirlpool metaphor to describe his catastrophic state. When in the whirlpool, he was panicked that his business would fail, which he would associate with being a "bad" person. The therapist and he identified certain interventions to avoid falling into a whirlpool. First, efforts were made to build a "platform" from which he could step back and view the whirlpool, reevaluating the catastrophic feelings relative to his actual situation. For example, the therapist and he were able to connect others not paying bills to his feeling ignored or unrecognized, as he did with his parents, rather than being an actual financial concern. Second was to review the record of his portfolio and business earnings; having a concrete representation of his actual success aided him in challenging these catastrophic experiences and representations. A third approach was to bring to mind how he was using these funds to support others. The notion of having a "legacy" helped him strengthen the emotional link to others he helped in his life and their appreciation of him, challenging the view of himself as "bad."

These shifts were reflected in changes in the transference, further aiding the relief of depressive feelings and catastrophic states. Rather than anticipating negative judgments from the therapist, he began to experience him as more supportive and collaborative. In fact, he began to rib the therapist about his own value, jokingly asking for refunds for what he saw as educating him about business matters. This helped to provide a way to more effectively express his anger through using humor.

WORKING THROUGH IN PrFPP: MR. M

Further information about triggers of problems: Therapist and patient recognized how delays in payment were misperceived as catastrophic, as he felt ignored by others. He also became more aware of how bullying others in business would trigger guilt and feelings of being a bad person.

Increased understanding of developmental history and its impact on current perceptions and problems: He developed a further understanding of how his sense of badness related to the emotional unresponsiveness and judgmental attitudes of his parents, as business was the only thing he was perceived as being good at. Therefore, perceived "failures" in business led him back to catastrophic feelings of "badness."

Ongoing addressing/confronting problematic self and other representations: The therapist and he increasingly confronted his self-view of being bad with a focus on his support of others and others being appreciative of him, creating feelings of being good that did not derive from business successes alone.

Further addressing areas of conflict, problematic defenses: He recognized that anger at himself for being bad stemmed in part from anger at his parents becoming self-directed, along with wanting to maintain attachment to them by accepting the "bad" role.

Identifying mentalization impairments and building mentalization skills: Therapist and patient recognized that his mentalization skills were restricted by negative views of others as judgmental or unresponsive rather than identifying them as having their own vulnerabilities. He increasingly realized how an understanding of others enabled him to approach them in different ways, including positively, aiding his success.

Ongoing use of the transference: Rather than continuing to view the therapist as judgmental, he shifted toward seeing the relationship as more collaborative, sometimes ribbing the therapist, asking for a discount when he provided information about how businesses worked.

Shifts in behavior—anger management: As his anger diminished and his understanding of his children's issues increased, he shifted toward a more collaborative, positive stance toward them. This change led to a more positive relationship, an increased ability to help them and a greater appreciation from them, further easing his feelings of being a "bad" person.

Ongoing development of skills to address problems: Therapist and patient worked on building a "platform" to avoid falling into a "whirlpool," working to recognize that the actual state of his business affairs was not catastrophic. This effort occurred in part by identifying concrete information that demonstrated his financial stability and by recognizing his caring for others. In addition, it was important to understand that problems with his business did not make him a "bad person."

MS. EE'S SELF-LOATHING

Ms. EE, discussed in Chapter 7, described a resurgence of self-attacks in the 2 weeks preceding her session. The therapist viewed this resurgence as an opportunity to further expand their understanding of contributing psychodynamic factors and reduce her vulnerability to episodes of self-loathing. When exploring triggers, she notably reported an increase in assertiveness during that time period, expressing stronger views about what steps to take in her mother's care, including to her brother. Her input and firm opinions were based on a greater understanding of her mother's issues that stemmed from her academic knowledge.

However, a few days after she expressed her views, she experienced an intense backlash of guilt, seeing herself as having been too aggressive and damaging in putting her ideas forward. Her mother and brother had become angry at the strength of her suggestions and devalued them, and Ms. EE accepted this family mythology. She suddenly felt that she was incompetent in helping others and did not deserve care herself, stating she had no right to complain when "people were suffering in war zones." She attacked herself for being "too opinionated."

THERAPIST: It seems as if you're having a backlash reaction to your newfound assertiveness. It's not clear what the problem is in expressing your views about your mother's care. But your responses triggered a lot of guilt and accepting the family's attitudes that you're somehow bad or incompetent.

Ms. EE: That makes sense about the backlash. It felt like this self-loathing had come out of nowhere, but I have been asserting myself more. Maybe I think I should be put back in my place.

THERAPIST: You shift back to a view in which you see yourself as bad and deserving of being attacked, and unfortunately your family is happy to play that role. And you inadvertently do it to yourself. At the same time, you feel as if you're not allowed to take care of yourself.

MS. EE: Doesn't that make sense to be chastised if I'm bad? I'm supposed to be helping my mother, and I'm not really doing it.

THERAPIST: That's not really clear, as when you were in your assertive mode you really felt it was important for your mother to take the steps you were suggesting. But even if somehow those steps were not correct, it's difficult to understand the extent to which you attack yourself.

MS. EE: You're right. It kind of doesn't make sense.

THERAPIST: Only in your negative mode in which somehow you accept that you could never do the right thing or enough for your mother. And that you don't deserve to take care of yourself, as you should be taking care of others.

MS. EE: When you view it like that, it's really sad that I would feel that way. And now I'm understanding it again, back in mode A, recognizing that I'm too harsh, whereas in my negative mode B, I can't see my way out.

Ms. EE increasingly made use of the therapist's description of mode A, in which her self-view was relatively benign, and mode B, in which she was intensely self-critical, to help her recognize the degree and unfairness of her self-loathing. Being able to articulate these modes helped her to identify when she began to shift from mode A to mode B and consider how and why this was occurring. This process was helpful because once she was in mode B it was hard to see her way out or recognize her negativity. As noted in Chapter 2, this kind of split in self and other representations and affects is not uncommon in the case of individuals who experienced significant trauma early in their lives that included abuse and/or neglect. The internalization of the view of the self as bad, damaging, or undeserving can interfere with being able to adopt or consider a more benign self-representation. This negative state and/or self-loathing can stem from (1) an internalization of this representation from caregivers; (2) anger at caregivers that causes conflict and is directed inward; and/or (3) a need to maintain a relationship by accepting abuse because it is the only relationship possible.

WORKING THROUGH MR. FF'S AVOIDANT BEHAVIOR

With further exploration, it emerged that Mr. FF, discussed in Chapter 7, had been increasingly constricted in his lifestyle, spending most of his time outside of work watching television and cooking. The therapist and Mr. FF realized how resistant he would become if others asked him to do something different from his usual daily routines. He behaved in a "passive–aggressive" manner, essentially refusing to do the alternate activity suggested by his husband or son. In exploring these routines, it became evident they had an important protective function, as considering any change felt dangerous, typically causing him significant distress. The therapist worked with him to identify the basis of these fears. For example, it became clear that he was more anxious than he had admitted previously about social activities, feeling he would be viewed as inadequate and not successful enough.

As he described the safety of his routines and the level of threat in disrupting them, he recalled feeling protected in his room from his father's temperamental and judgmental episodes. His father's outbursts were unpredictable and sometimes included physical and verbal abuse. Thus, he spent hours in his bedroom playing video games or studying, rarely going out to spend time with family except when his father was absent. The therapist worked to identify with Mr. FF that this danger was no longer present, as he acknowledged that, although there were tensions between himself and his husband, Albert did not attack him in the way that his father had.

However, it became clear that his resistance to doing new activities did not just take the form of passive aggression. Albert confronted him about angry outbursts he had apparently minimized and asked Mr. FF to discuss them in therapy; apparently, he would become furious when Albert pressed him to do something different from his usual routine. It emerged that he avoided discussing his temperamental episodes because he found them embarrassing, as they reminded him of his father. After becoming enraged, he would experience a wave of guilt.

The therapist worked to help him understand his angry feelings, so he might better cope with them. Partly, he was angry that his husband pressed him to confront the threat he experienced in making changes. Furthermore, when his son and Albert pressured him, or went out without him, he felt furious about being "ganged up on" by them. He became irritated toward his son for constantly challenging him about his inhibitions and other matters, stating that his son believed he was correct about everything. He became aware that his son's "know-it-all" attitude reminded him of his father. Indeed, he experienced the pressure from Albert and his son as akin to his father's bullying and controlling behavior.

Understanding the developmental origins of his temper episodes helped him to better control them. His anger eased further as, with increased mentalization, he was able to better recognize the frustration these restrictions caused for his husband and son. Rather than simply pressuring him, they very much hoped he would spend more time with them. The understanding of the misperceptions of their behavior helped to reduce his resistance to trying new activities.

With this shift in mind, the therapist encouraged the patient to take steps to try new pursuits despite his resistance. Indeed, Mr. FF acknowledged that, when he went to plays or museums, he enjoyed them despite feeling pressured to abandon his routine at home. The social fears of judgment were also found to relate to his father's judgmental attitudes, as the ridicule he anticipated was similar. This awareness enabled him to challenge his social anxiety, and he was able to take pleasure in some social activities. The therapist made a point of contrasting his anticipated fears to his actual enjoyment of going outside of his routine. Using these approaches, he steadily expanded the range of events he attended with his husband and son.

TERMINATION

The next chapter describes the termination phase in PrFPP. In some instances, a termination date is set based on a predetermined number of sessions. In its more open-ended form, at a certain point the therapist and patient assess that a significant degree of reduction of problems has occurred, along with working through vulnerabilities to recurrence, enabling termination to take place. The following chapter discusses how to make such a determination and productively use the termination period to maintain and further treatment gains. This process includes addressing the patient's feelings and fantasies regarding the therapist in the context of ending treatment. Therapist and patient work to summarize vulnerabilities to recurrence and interventions and skills designed to address them.

> ### QUESTIONS AND IDEAS TO THINK ABOUT
>
> 1. Discuss with some of your patients how they see their progress in the treatment. With which problems do they see themselves as making progress? What have they understood about those problems or learned to handle differently? What problems are the patients still struggling with? Consider ideas for how to address those persistent problems.
>
> 2. With one of your patients, try the exercise of holding back on impulsive behavior for 30 minutes. What thoughts, feelings, and urges did the patient experience? Were any behaviors effective in preventing them from acting on their urges? What did you and the patient learn from this exercise?

WORKSHEET 8.1
Elements of Working Through Problems

These questions will help organize your understanding about the sources of your problems. They will also help you and your therapist evaluate the progress you are making in addressing your problems.

What information can you provide about the triggers of your problems?

What kinds of things have you recognized from your past that have an impact on your problems?

How have you addressed or confronted your views of self or others that have added to your problems?

How have you addressed feelings and wishes that you struggle with, and how have you tried to manage them?

(continued)

From *Skills Training in Psychodynamic Psychotherapy*, by Fredric N. Busch. Copyright © 2026 The Guilford Press. Permission to photocopy this worksheet, or to download and print additional copies (www.guilford.com/busch-forms), is granted to purchasers of this book for personal use or use with clients; see copyright page for details.

Elements of Working Through Problems (page 2 of 2)

Can you identify faulty expectations of others, and if so, how have you adjusted these expectations?

How has your view toward your therapist shifted over the course of treatment?

How have you noticed your behavior changing when working through your problems?

What kinds of skills have you developed to address your problems?

WORKSHEET 8.2

Holding Back on Impulsive Behaviors

Please hold off on your impulsive behaviors (e.g., drug or alcohol use, shopping, sexual behavior, etc.) for 30 minutes. During this time, write down the thoughts, feelings, and urges that come to mind. Also try certain thoughts or actions (e.g., exercise, calling a friend) that may help relieve the urges to pursue these behaviors. Please note these activities and their effectiveness in managing your impulses.

Thoughts:

Feelings:

Urges:

Thoughts or actions to relieve urges:

Please note whether these thoughts or actions were helpful in relieving urges:

From *Skills Training in Psychodynamic Psychotherapy*, by Fredric N. Busch. Copyright © 2026 The Guilford Press. Permission to photocopy this worksheet, or to download and print additional copies (*www.guilford.com/busch-forms*), is granted to purchasers of this book for personal use or use with clients; see copyright page for details.

CHAPTER 9

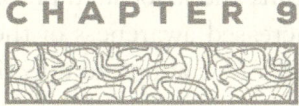

Termination

PrFPP includes the value of exploring the patient's reactions to the end of treatment found in any psychodynamic psychotherapy but combines it with a more structured approach to evaluating the patient's progress and the development of skills to address problems post treatment (Busch, 2022). In some circumstances, a termination date is set based on a predetermined number of sessions. In the more open-ended form of PrFPP, the therapist and patient assess when a significant degree of reduction of problems has occurred, along with working through vulnerabilities to recurrence, enabling termination to take place. This chapter discusses how to make such a determination and productively use the termination period to maintain and further treatment gains. Termination also includes addressing the patient's feelings and fantasies regarding the therapist in the context of ending treatment, as in more traditional psychodynamic psychotherapy. However, in PrFPP these transference dynamics are specifically related to problem areas and their vulnerability to recurrence. The therapist and patient can use guiding questions in session or worksheets to summarize progress on problems, dynamic vulnerabilities to recurrence, and helpful interventions and skills designed to address them.

ASSESSING THE PATIENT'S DEGREE OF IMPROVEMENT

An important task in identifying readiness for ending treatment is assessing the degree of relief of the patient's problems. This determination is based upon the level of change and working through, and the degree to which the problem appears vulnerable to recurrence. For example, with anxiety disorder patients, improvement is evidenced by a significant reduction in the patient's symptoms and associated problematic behaviors, such as avoidance and unassertiveness, an increased awareness of the nature of anxiety triggers and psychodynamic contributors, and a new ability to effectively manage the challenges and emotions brought up by stressors.

In addition, there is a focus on clarifying and furthering the development of **psychodynamic skills** that patients use to help address persistent problems and the potential for recurrence. Although behavioral changes are not typically considered a psychodynamic skill, in this treatment these shifts are recognized as important to change and as addressing contributory psychodynamic factors. Psychodynamic skills include:

1. The capacity to identify contexts and emotions likely to exacerbate problems and to employ interventions to address these triggers.
2. The capacity to identify and address the impact of the developmental history on problems.
3. The ability to identify and confront contributory negative self and other representations.
4. The ability to recognize and manage conflicted feelings and fantasies that exacerbate problems.
5. The use of mentalization skills to help address adverse perceptions of others that contribute to problems.
6. The employment of behavioral changes to better manage intrapsychic and interpersonal conflict.

It can be of value for the therapist and patients to make a more formal assessment of the development of psychodynamic skills targeting problems derived from the psychodynamic formulation. An advantage of patients conceptualizing these dynamics and interventions is to describe them in ways that are comprehensible and meaningful to them. This exercise also gives an opportunity to think through and formulate the skills they have learned and discuss them with the therapist. Finally, patients can refer back to this formulation in order to refresh their memories of what they have understood about their problems and the means of addressing them, even after termination. They can also work on using these skills to address new issues that emerge in their lives.

Below is an approach to this part of the termination process. With this approach, you can assess the patient's understanding of the formulation of their problems and the development of these skills. Worksheet 9.1: Psychodynamic Skills to Address Problems and Their Potential Recurrence (pp. 211–212; all worksheets available online at *www.guilford.com/busch-forms*) is a handy tool for doing this work. The therapist can either hand the worksheet to patients to fill out on their own, and then discuss their answers in a subsequent session, or the therapist can fill it out with the patient, asking them guiding questions. Sample answers are given in the case of Mr. F below.

CASE EXAMPLE: MR. F'S WORKAHOLISM

As described previously (Chapter 2), Mr. F felt pressured to take on additional clients, even though his business was full, and he struggled to complete the tasks that were required by his clientele. Notable triggers included calls from potential clients requesting his services, to which he felt pressured to respond despite his recognition that he could barely manage his current tasks. His focus on work also caused conflicts with his wife due to his being less available to her and the children. He had tried to manage his stress by developing a flirtation with his administrator and drinking nightly to relieve anxiety. The therapist and the patient explored the nature of the urges Mr. F felt to accept new clients. These factors included a sense that he had a responsibility to take care of them, even though they were not yet his clients. A second contributor was the pressure he felt to achieve and make money based on his father's opinion of what made a person worthy. A third was worries that he had about his financial situation if he did not take on the client, despite being financially stable.

With PrFPP, the patient was increasingly able to interrupt his tendency to add new clients when overworked by challenging these notions and pressures. One aid was recognizing that he did not yet owe anything to these clients, so it was not necessary to take them on. Indeed, he understood this sense of pressure stemmed in part from his need to attend to his "emotionally needy" mother when growing up, sometimes canceling get-togethers with friends or dates in order to do so. A second area was to challenge his father's focus on making money and achieving by recognizing other values that were of importance to him, such as spending time with his wife and children. In therapy, he became more aware of the adverse impact on him of his father's frequent absences from the home to pursue professional achievement, as well as his own sense of being "an afterthought" in terms of his father's interests. Finally, he addressed how his financial worries were overstated, contributed to by his father's focus on making money.

By keeping these factors in mind, he was typically, though not always, able to turn down new clients. Through these behavioral changes, his work became less demanding, though still busy, requiring less time in the evenings and on weekends. His anxiety eased as he felt less pressure to keep up with an excessive workload. His capacity to be at home more helped relieve tensions and conflicts with his wife. Indeed, Mr. F had interpreted his wife's criticisms of him as attempts to undermine him and a lack of recognition of the time his work required. However, through mentalization efforts, he became more accepting of the idea that his wife missed him during his absences and was frustrated by the greater responsibilities she had for the children.

Their relationship shifted in a more positive direction, and this change along with diminished pressure reduced the intensity of the flirtation he had with his administrator. He also believed the therapist disapproved of his flirtation, which had continued, though less intensely, seeing it as a betrayal of his wife. The therapist noted that, although he had not pronounced judgment about his behavior, Mr. F himself had felt guilty about it. Perhaps he was projecting? The patient felt that that made sense and recognized his persistent guilt about his interactions with the administrator. A more professional stance with her helped ease some of the guilt. Although he remained friendly with her and sometimes flirtatious, he no longer talked with her about his wish to be more intimate. Furthermore, he recognized that the flirtation had given him a sense of power and impact that helped overcome feelings of inadequacy related to his father and his presumptive lack of achievement.

In the context of diminishing anxiety, the therapist worked with Mr. F to reduce his drinking. An initial goal was decreasing his use from three to two drinks per night. As he felt less stress and worry about his workload, he felt less of an urge to drink to relieve his anxiety. He was able to reduce his drinking on weeknights, although he missed getting the "buzz" that he would experience with three drinks. They then set a further goal of not drinking on three nights per week. The therapist suggested using Worksheet 8.2: Holding Back on Impulsive Behaviors (see Chapter 8), which Mr. F would utilize to monitor the feelings that emerged when he held off on drinking. They began with having him wait 30 minutes past his usual start time.

The therapist and the patient found that, when he delayed or held off on drinking, as well as when he was not as busy at work as he hoped, he confronted stretches in which he felt bored, inadequate, or sad. The feelings of inadequacy were addressed as a new problem; the therapist commented that their emergence was a sign of progress, as he had avoided them through compensatory overwork, flirting, and drinking. They explored this problem, determining that it represented in part his reaction to feeling that his father was not interested in or approving of him if he was not constantly busy or successful enough. They recognized the importance of him learning to tolerate these feelings and find other areas of interest; he began to search for more alternative activities. He took up golf, having played it in years previously, which he enjoyed with friends and could also use as a way to be in contact with clients. Also, the camaraderie he experienced with others on the golf course helped address his feelings of inadequacy. The therapist and the patient recognized that having a group of friends, which he previously did not have time for, helped him feel better about himself and reduce his anxiety.

A sense of inadequacy emerged in the transference in the context of discussing termination. He experienced feelings of rejection by the therapist, as if they were stopping because he was not as interested as he felt with his father. The therapist pointed out the link of these rejected feelings and reminded him that the termination plan was a mutual decision. In addition, he was angry at the therapist because these feelings of inadequacy, like many of his problems, persisted to a degree, as initially he hoped for a "cure" of his difficulties. At the same time, he was able to recognize and mourn the limits of therapy, realizing that some struggle with psychological and emotional issues was part of life.

Below is the list of problems that the therapist and Mr. F created, all of which had demonstrated a marked reduction at the time of this assessment:

Problem list

1. Compulsive working

   Mr. F was now able to turn down enough new clients to avoid working most evenings and weekends.

2. Generalized anxiety

   Mr. F's anxiety eased significantly, as he no longer felt under intense pressure to complete work tasks.

3. Conflicts with his wife

   Conflicts with his wife diminished, as Mr. F was able to be at home and available to his family most nights and weekends.

4. Alcohol use

   Mr. F was able to reduce alcohol use in part due to reduced work pressure.

5. Underlying feelings of inadequacy

   As Mr. F reduced his drinking, feelings of inadequacy emerged that eased in the context of the changes he made in his workload and in not feeling judged by the therapist.

Below are the answers that Mr. F provided on his worksheet:

Psychodynamic Skills to Address Problems and Their Potential Recurrence

Are you able to notice when your problems are being triggered? Can you identify and address the situations and feelings that contribute to this?

I'm aware that I still have urges to take on new clients, even when I have too much work. I recognize that it's driven by feeling inadequate at some level and needing to achieve, and that I feel I have to respond to others' needs. I've been able to use this information to turn down some new clients, which helped ease my workload.

Are you able to recognize and work with how your past contributes to your problems?

I realize now that my tendency to overwork and pressure to achieve are related to seeking my father's approval, who was a difficult man to impress. I also understand that my tendencies are stronger because I felt pressure to care for my mother. I'm able to use this information to steer myself away from overworking, though it's not always easy. I want to make choices that are good for me and not be chasing after my father's approval, which may have been impossible to get. I recognize that, when I'm starting to get anxious, I probably have too much work to do and should turn down cases.

Are you able to identify and address how your views and expectations of yourself and others contribute to your problems?

I recognize that I've had an overly negative view of myself and my accomplishments, and this was likely related to my father's excessively high expectations. I'm also able to feel better about myself now that I've made changes in my life, such as having more time with my wife and family. In addition to feeling that others will judge me for my lack of achievement, I tend to believe that they can't manage without me. I recognize that if I can't work with them, they'll just find another accountant!

Do you recognize how conflicts about feelings and wishes contribute to your problems? How is this helpful?

I've learned that I've been mad at my father for having unreasonable expectations and not being more supportive of me. Because he couldn't tolerate any anger toward him, I think I suppressed it and directed it toward myself. I try to think about this when I get self-critical. I also think I've indirectly expressed my anger by rebelling. I have an attitude toward my wife that she's not going to control me, and I rebel with overwork, drinking, and flirting, but that doesn't help me improve my life.

How have your misunderstandings of others' feelings and expectations contributed to your problems? How do you address these misconceptions?

I realize how I anticipate that others are going to be judgmental of me or that I think they will be unable to function without my help. I sometimes interpret others as being judgmental when they're not. I now try to be alert to this tendency. Also, I recognize that other people, besides my family, can survive without my help.

What behavioral changes have you found helpful in dealing with your problems?

It's clear to me that turning down cases brings me relief and that my drinking and flirtation have been attempts to deal with these pressures and rebel. Although I'm drawn toward these behaviors, I understand that they lead to more difficulties and distress.

CASE EXAMPLE: MS. J'S SHOPPING COMPULSION

As Ms. J made further progress in controlling her shopping impulses, she was able to manage them enough to stop herself from going into additional debt. She had a better recognition of the triggers of her shopping in terms of feeling deprived and angry and was able to challenge those urges through exercise and contacting a friend. There were ongoing tensions with her husband Tom, who remained frustrated that they were in debt from the patient's prior spending. Ms. J continued to be angered by her husband's attitude toward her, feeling that he should be more empathic to her struggles. There were also tensions when Ms. J requested money from Tom to pay off the debt. Although his family had resources, he wanted to be independent and was reluctant to ask for help. Despite these persistent struggles, Ms. J and her husband still enjoyed each other's company and liked similar activities. Although the therapist suggested couples counseling, Ms. J did not think it would be necessary. Her anxiety and anger eased as she contained her spending and better managed her feelings of deprivation.

Work in the transference intensified as the therapist broached the topic of termination. Ms. J experienced ending treatment as a form of abandonment not unlike what she experienced with her mother. The therapist recognized how she might perceive it this way given the traumatic impact of her mother's abandonment but assured her that this was a decision they would make together; the therapist had no intention of unilaterally ending her treatment. In PrFPP with a set termination date, the therapist would approach this differently, exploring the feelings while reminding the patient that the termination date was set at the beginning of treatment for specific reasons (e.g., as part of a clinic protocol). With Ms. J, her reaction provided further opportunities to identify her vulnerability to feeling abandoned and to be alert to the ongoing impact of these fears.

For instance, Ms. J reported that she intermittently worried that her husband might suddenly decide to leave her, something she had not previously revealed. However, Tom had never brought up such wishes or made reference to such a plan, even when he was at his angriest with the patient. The therapist reassured her that this possibility seemed highly unlikely and could readily be ascribed to her fears of abandonment. In fact, Ms. J acknowledged that one of the significant reasons she married Tom, despite certain frustrations with him, was his loyalty and commitment as a partner. The recognition that these fears were related to her traumatic experiences with her mother helped reduce her worries that Tom would leave her.

The therapist reviewed her problem list and the significant improvement in her problems:

Problem List

1. Shopping compulsion

   The patient managed to control her impulses adequately to stop increasing her debt.

2. Anxiety disorder

   The patient's symptoms of intense anxiety eased, as she was better able to manage her shopping.

3. Conflicts with her husband

   Conflicts with her husband diminished, as she gained better control of her shopping compulsion and financial situation and better understood his concerns.

When the therapist suggested that Ms. J fill out Worksheet 9.1 (pp. 211–212) to describe the formulation and skills she gained, she responded that she would prefer that the therapist fill it out for them to discuss. The therapist explored Ms. J's hesitancy, which was related to fears that she would appear unintelligent in her answers. However, as she continued to express discomfort, he also agreed to move the process forward by completing it. Ms. J reviewed the therapist's responses (see below) and expressed her strong agreement with them.

Psychodynamic Skills to Address Problems and Their Potential Recurrence

Are you able to notice when your problems are being triggered? Can you identify and address the situations and feelings that contribute to this?

You've been able to recognize that your urges to shop are triggered when you feel angry or deprived, or sometimes rejected. You've developed ways to step back and manage these urges before you start shopping. You've identified interventions, such as contacting others or exercising, to further reduce these urges.

Are you able to recognize and work with how your past contributes to your problems?

You've been better able to recognize how your experience of being abandoned by your mother, and the subsequent reduction of contact as well as financial losses, contributed to you feeling deprived, angry, and wanting to shop to feel better. You've learned to keep this in mind to better wrestle with these urges.

Are you able to identify and address how your views and expectations of yourself and others contribute to your problems?

You've understood that you see yourself as deprived and prone to feeling rejected and others as not responsive and rejecting. But you've recognized that, in many ways, you're not deprived and that your husband, though frustrated with your shopping, is very responsive to you. You've used this information to challenge these negative views.

Do you recognize how conflicts about feelings and wishes contribute to your problems? How is this helpful?

You're aware now that you have trouble managing your anger or feelings of needing others and feel conflicted about them. You overly worried that your anger or needs would lead to abandonment. Your awareness has led to you better managing these emotions and feeling less threatened.

How have your misunderstandings of others' feelings and expectations contributed to your problems? How do you address these misconceptions?

You've tended to expect rejection or attack from others. This made it hard for you to recognize that your husband was actually very concerned about you, even though he was frustrated about your spending. You're able to keep this more in mind now that you recognize this tendency.

What behavioral changes have you found helpful in dealing with your problems?

You've cut down on your shopping, even though the urge is still there to act on your impulses, as you recognize that not spending eases your anxiety and conflict with your husband.

CASE EXAMPLE: MR. A'S PANIC ATTACKS

Mr. A had an ongoing reduction of panic attacks, as he increasingly addressed his conflicts around pressure to respond to others and his management of aloneness. In his efforts to confront others, he found unexpectedly that they were more responsive to direct communication of his feelings than he thought. He began to discuss with his husband and a friend about how to talk to them about frustrations he had. For instance, he got angry at his friend when the friend was pressuring him to accept a point of view on a topic Mr. A disagreed with. He said, "George, you stop talking to me like that!" However, instead of the friend getting angry at him, George responded, "Okay, well, at least you're telling me what you think." George explained that in his family that was how people communicated when they felt angry, and he was used to "people screaming at each other to get it out of their systems." He preferred it to Mr. A's indirect expression of anger or passive aggression. This greatly relieved Mr. A's feelings of anxiety and frustration.

In addition, Mr. A became increasingly comfortable in settings in which he had felt alone and anxious. He recognized when he had feelings of loneliness and that these feelings were not actually dangerous to him. This included situations when his husband was away, in which he had become aware that he simultaneously felt relieved to be separated from him and greatly missed him. In these contexts, he recognized that it sometimes helped him to contact others and arrange to spend time with them. However, he increasingly identified that he was able to enjoy time alone and could more readily focus on his writing. In addition, he became engaged by closely observing interactions between people on the street, and these observations gave him ideas for his writing.

As Mr. A felt safer with the dual concerns regarding pressure and separation from others, his panic attacks became increasingly uncommon. Instead, he experienced mild to moderate feelings of anxiety that he could use as signals to help him identify that he was in a situation that felt uncomfortable to him. He was able to recognize that, in some of these circumstances, he was feeling pressured by others and angry about it. One of these situations occurred with his son pressing him to get more exercise. He was able to say to his son, "I appreciate your concern and have considered what you're saying, but I have my own thoughts and ideas about what I want to do, and I'm trying to take care of myself. I respect your views and hope you can respect mine, but we might just agree to disagree about them." This led to his son raising his concerns less often, even though some tensions remained between them.

As noted in Chapter 8, Mr. A suspected that the therapist might, for his own reasons, want him to stay in therapy, mirroring his sense of being pressured by others' needs. However, he increasingly recognized that the therapist did not judge or criticize him when he needed to miss sessions, such as when he went on speaking engagements about his most recent book. These worries returned when he brought up that, given the reduction in his anxiety and panic attacks and better management of his relationships, he felt it would be worth trying to take a break from therapy. When the therapist stated that he agreed that this should be considered, the patient's anxiety diminished.

At that point, however, he had a surge of fear and sadness about missing the therapy and worried that he might have difficulty dealing with his problems alone. He had considered the treatment enormously helpful and would definitely miss the therapist's support. The therapist was able to link these feelings with his early life experiences of aloneness when he felt that his parents were not emotionally responsive. He also reassured the patient that he would be able to come back for treatment if he thought it was necessary. As part of termination, he worked with Mr. A in filling out the forms regarding his progress and the psychodynamic skills he developed (see below).

Problem list

1. Panic disorder

    These attacks were significantly reduced, although he had an occasional panic attack with unclear precipitants and anxiety in situations in which he felt pressured or alone.

2. Unassertiveness

    Mr. A became much more assertive with others in expressing his wishes with them, especially when he wanted space to himself.

3. Fears of aloneness

    Mr. A became able to recognize when he became lonely and ask for support from others. Additionally, he found that closely observing others relieved his loneliness and helped spur his writing.

Psychodynamic Skills to Address Problems and Their Potential Recurrence

Are you able to notice when your problems are being triggered? Can you identify and address the situations and feelings that contribute to this?

I have a pretty good idea of what triggers my panic episodes. This includes situations in which I'm pressured by others' demands or when I feel alone. I'm pretty understanding of these circumstances now and what to do about them. But there's still the occasional panic episode that's a bit of a mystery. It doesn't happen very often, and I can reassure myself with this knowledge.

Are you able to recognize and work with how your past contributes to your problems?

I understand how I got worried about feeling both alone emotionally and pressured growing up. It helps to be able to recognize where these problems came from, as I realize I'm not in the same position now and can take some steps to deal with it!

Are you able to identify and address how your views and expectations of yourself and others contribute to your problems?

I felt before that I didn't have a right to assert myself. Now I recognize that I can tell my friends or husband what my needs are. I used to expect that they'd be very hurt or angry if I said something about needing space. I've seen that this could happen, but other times, people seem to appreciate the feedback or information I give them. I also realized that, when I was alone, I thought there was nothing to be done about it. But now I recognize how I can contact others or engage in activities that help to relieve these feelings.

Do you recognize how conflicts about feelings and wishes contribute to your problems? How has this been helpful?

I had a prior therapist suggest that panic sometimes came from anger, but I hadn't quite understood that I feared my anger would hurt or enrage others. This probably has something to do with my father's temper, which was very scary. But I now realize that there are ways to modulate how I express it. Also, I think I was afraid to feel that I was lonely because I felt others wouldn't respond. Now I recognize when I have that feeling.

How have your misunderstandings of others' feelings and expectations contributed to your problems? How do you address these misconceptions?

I didn't expect others to react well to my expressing any kind of negative feelings toward them, whether it was anger or needing support from them. I don't think I even realized this. But inside, I anticipated that they would be angry, hurt, or unresponsive. Now I can think about what they're actually experiencing. Maybe they want to hear what I have to say, or maybe they want to help when I ask them.

What behavioral changes have you found helpful in dealing with your problems?

I recognize that it's important to address tensions with others rather than keep them to myself or express them indirectly. I also know that, when I'm alone, it's good to try to connect with others or just go exploring the city.

CASE EXAMPLE: MS. GG'S OVERRESPONSIBILITY AND DEPRESSION

Ms. GG increasingly noticed her tendency to take on responsibilities that were not hers and made efforts to avoid these situations. She became aware that, when she did accept these tasks, she would become depressed because she felt overwhelmed by the responsibilities involved and could not find a way to reduce them. She became alert to guilty feelings that drove both her acceptance of responsibility and her difficulty reducing her workload once she was involved.

With this increased awareness, she and the therapist were able to identify another area of risk: pressure to take care of her stepfather, who was dealing with increasing health problems. These tasks involved taking him to doctors' appointments and arranging care for him at home. In exploring her attitude toward caring for him, it emerged that he had closer family members who could step in to help with these problems. Additionally, she revealed that her mother was not close to him at the time of her death. Although this set of tasks had not reached the degree of disrupting her life, it was putting her at risk. As she recognized that she was drawn into responsibilities that were not hers, she began discussions with his family members about taking over his care.

Given her increased capacities to reduce and avert new tasks and pressures, she and the therapist began to discuss termination. She felt sad about leaving therapy and realized that she had felt more isolated from friends since she had spent so much time on her business responsibilities. Additionally, she had become more isolated during the pandemic. However, she was hesitant to reengage with her friends, and in this context, a previously unidentified problem emerged—social anxiety. She noted how she had always been fearful about social situations, although these fears tended to be relieved when a friendship became close. However, as she was separated from her friends during the pandemic, these fears reemerged.

In exploring these worries, her concerns focused on either being seen as "stupid" or saying the wrong things. She described a history of worries about her intelligence from when she was very young. She recalled being held back in first grade and in fifth grade being assigned to the basic, rather than the advanced, math class. Her father was also highly focused on intelligence as an admired characteristic and tended to be highly judgmental of the patient and others. He would get irritated when Ms. GG did not quickly grasp what he was communicating. Although her successful career helped her overcome these fears, they would reemerge in unfamiliar social situations.

THERAPIST: I think it would be helpful to challenge your social anxiety. We know that you really didn't have these fears with your friends prior to the pandemic and becoming absorbed in the business. What occurs to you as you think of these worries now?

MS. GG: I think in part it's feeling out of practice. I haven't been getting together with others except on Zoom. And then I think I worry I don't have much of interest to say. I used to go to plays and movies and read more, so I had something to discuss. Now with all this work, I feel like I've become a boring person.

THERAPIST: Hopefully, now that your family is going to sell the business, you'll have more time to read things and, with the pandemic ending, more chances to go out. But your friends never seemed to think you weren't intelligent.

MS. GG: No. It's probably more inside of me. I agree I should probably set up some activities, and it will probably go fine. Also, I should start reading again. I really enjoyed doing that, and it's for the most part been sidelined.

Given her current isolation, she and the therapist decided to delay termination for 3 months while she made what turned out to be successful efforts to reengage with her friends. As this effort proceeded, the therapist further explored self-esteem issues involving concerns about her intelligence. This led to the recognition that she believed that her "not being smart enough" contributed to her father's lack of interest in her. However, she realized in exploring this perception that her father's distance related to a more general lack of interest in his children. He was very focused on his professional success and paid little more attention to her older brother, who was a straight A student and viewed as very bright. It emerged that another factor that motivated her in the family business was a wish to demonstrate her capability of managing it, though in actuality no one questioned her competence.

Here is Ms. GG's problem list and the therapist's notes on the progress she had made on each of them:

Problem list

1. Depression
   The patient's depressive symptoms significantly improved as she became less busy with her work and more involved with friends, except for occasional down periods when she still felt isolated.
2. Overresponsibility
   She became more alert to internal pressures to take on tasks that were not required of her and felt some freeing from pressures associated with them.

3. Guilt

    The patient's propensity to guilty feelings went beyond the association with her depression and included both pressure to care for others and conflicts with anger. As she better understood these factors, there was a reduction of her tendency toward guilty feelings, which also helped ease her overresponsibility.

4. Social anxiety and isolation

    These problems, recognized late in the treatment, diminished significantly as the patient recognized her fears that others found her uninteresting were excessive.

5. Fear of inadequacy

    The patient recognized that she had fears about her intelligence stemming from her childhood experiences that contributed to her social anxiety and overresponsibility. Acknowledging her capability and intelligence helped her further ease these problems (see below).

Psychodynamic Skills to Address Problems and Their Potential Recurrence

Are you able to notice when your problems are being triggered? Can you identify and address the situations and feelings that contribute to this?

I'm really alert to my tendency to take on tasks that I don't really have to. I don't want what happened with the business to happen again. I'm aware that I start to feel guilty and pressured and recognize that if I do so, I could end up depressed again.

Are you able to recognize and work with how your past contributes to your problems?

I've understood that the expectation for me to take care of my mother as an adolescent was a contributor to my guilt and overresponsibility. Also, my father's limited interest in me, other than as a caretaker, added to feelings of inadequacy and concerns about my intellect.

Are you able to identify and address how your views and expectations of yourself and others contribute to your problems?

I've had the tendency to feel that I was somehow causing others pain and that it was my job to help them out. I also saw myself as uninteresting to others, except as it involved taking care of them. Now I work to challenge these views when I have them, recognizing that, with my friends, it's a give and take of our needs and wishes.

Do you recognize how conflicts about feelings and wishes contribute to your problems? How has this been helpful?

I've understood that I was really angry about the position I was put in by my parents at the same time that I felt terrible for my mother. Somehow, I turned that anger toward myself and viewed myself as the guilty, responsible party. It's been important to become more aware of my anger, such as toward family members who were happy to leave me to do the work.

How have your misunderstandings of others' feelings and expectations contributed to your problems? How do you address these misconceptions?

I've tended to think that others expected me to take care of jobs for them or that otherwise they wouldn't be interested in me. But now I understand that, although they're happy for me to take them on, they don't expect it. And my friends are just interested in being with me. I guess my father's attitude continued to have a big impact, and I wasn't aware of it.

What behavioral changes have you found helpful in dealing with your problems?

In some ways, it's keeping away from certain behaviors, like taking on new chores. I keep focused on getting together with my friends or engaging in other activities I enjoy.

RETURN TO TREATMENT

No therapy is 100% successful, and psychological or emotional problems are part of life. The therapist works with the patient to recognize these limitations and spend some time applying the skills they have developed to manage their problems as well as they can. Nevertheless, it is not unusual for patients to seek follow-up to cope with recurrence of problems or development of a new problem. Patients who received traditional psychodynamic psychotherapy sometimes have trouble clarifying what a prior therapy did or did not achieve and how it was helpful to them or not. In PrFPP, efforts are made to detail the patient's understanding of the origins of and skills to manage their problems in a formulation and worksheets. In the event of a recurrence or new problems, this knowledge helps the therapist and the patient explore the ways in which their skills were ineffective, how their vulnerabilities overrode the use of their skills, or in what ways the psychodynamic formulation needed to be modified. Frequently, a new stressor has overwhelmed the capacities and skills they achieved and requires an adjustment in their self-understanding and approaches to problems.

CASE EXAMPLE: MR. M'S STRUGGLE WITH ILLNESS

Mr. M, who had wrestled with depression and catastrophic fears regarding his business, terminated following the significant understanding and resolution of his fears, as described in Chapter 8. However, he returned 6 years later in an anxious and depressed state following a diagnosis of Parkinson's disease. Mr. M showed little in the way of neurological symptoms other than a tremor. Curiously, he was much more focused on the computers at his business being hacked than his Parkinson's. He was fearful and preoccupied that somehow the hack was going to disrupt his business or that some impropriety would be revealed that would get him into trouble. His sleep was disrupted, he was distracted from his work, and he was having trouble enjoying his usual activities.

A review of the impact of the hack on office computers was being conducted at the time, and so far, no significant damage had been found. In addition, Mr. M had few improprieties at his work that could get him into trouble, other than some borderline decisions regarding tax loopholes that had been approved by his accountant. He was also fearful that his competitor had been behind the hacking to get information, such as a client list, regarding the business. Although the therapist considered the possibility that the patient was bordering on delusions from the Parkinson's, it was clear that a hack of some significance had occurred, and Mr. M was able to reality test his fears of the entire business being disrupted, him getting into trouble, or his competitor having been involved.

Mr. M had always touted how fit he was despite his age, and the therapist knew Parkinson's would be a significant blow to his self-esteem. The therapist believed that the primary source of Mr. M's resurgence in anxiety about his business collapsing was related to his learning about his Parkinson's diagnosis:

THERAPIST: It's very curious that you're so focused on the computer hack, even though you've been reassured recently that there's no major damage, and that you've expressed little concern about the Parkinson's diagnosis.

MR. M: You know how I am. My worries about the business always come back.

THERAPIST: But that was usually when there was some degree of downturn in the business. And overall, you were managing those fears much better at the end of therapy. I'm wondering if this has more to do with the Parkinson's diagnosis than you realize.

MR. M: I guess that's possible. I mean, I don't have many symptoms. I know it can get bad; I'm hoping to avoid that by keeping in shape, but I know that doesn't always work.

THERAPIST: In a way, the Parkinson's feels like the hack: something that came out of nowhere, causes damage, and is intrusive.

MR. M: That is interesting. Maybe I should talk more about it?

As the therapist encouraged exploration of the impact of Parkinson's, Mr. M began to recognize more of his fears of debilitation and steadily became less focused on the hack. Partly, he was worried that his symptoms would interfere with his work functioning, which he still greatly enjoyed and was an important aspect of his identity. The therapist also investigated his fears of something "bad" being found about him through the hack that would cause him to get into trouble and its relationship to childhood fears. The patient then revealed that he had worried he had done something "wrong" in his management of his health that had caused the Parkinson's despite being assured that this was not the case. This perception could also be related to his fears of being back in his childhood traumatic situation.

His symptoms had been improving when he suddenly became very preoccupied with his tremor, which had worsened since the time of diagnosis. He began to believe that others were noticing the tremor and were judgmental of him about it. In particular, he was worried that clients would see him as impaired despite there being no change in his functioning and capacities at work. The therapist again linked this to his sense of being "bad" and others criticizing him on that basis. He also noted that this was a direct concern about his Parkinson's rather than the indirect fear as expressed with the computer hack. Such worries about Parkinson's made sense given the uncertainty of the course of the illness, but the catastrophic level of concern and the fears of rejection related to the patient's developmental trauma and its impact on his psyche.

As he became more tolerant of addressing his illness, he raised fears of death. Although his fears were comprehensible given his aging, exploration revealed that the threat of abandonment contributed to them. In that regard, he imagined death as a final rejection by others. This component of his fears was linked to the emotional disregard and judgment of his parents. Reminders about his sense of legacy and the way he was valued by his family helped ease these fears, though not entirely.

After several additional sessions, his anxiety about the tremor began to decrease, as the therapist's interpretations made sense to him, and he became aware that it was having little impact on his business or social life. He stated that he was ready to try being on his own again, with a request to return if there were further problems. He expressed appreciation of the therapist's help and support and felt that he had internalized the therapist's supportive view of him. He half-jokingly commented that the therapist would miss him, including his educational comments about business. The therapist confirmed that he would indeed miss the patient, that he had learned quite a bit from him and appreciated the opportunity to work with him.

As the therapist and patient had ready access to the formulation and interventions that had been helpful in his psychotherapeutic treatment, they were able to rapidly address the concerns brought on by the onset of his illness. Mr. M was quickly able to grasp these dynamics, which made sense to him, as his skills had been temporarily upended by this significant stressor. The approach of PrFPP had been particularly valuable for him. As with some other patients, he reminded the therapist at his last session that his two prior psychotherapies had not been nearly as effective. He had found the interventions of this treatment particularly helpful in relieving his distress and giving him an increased understanding of his vulnerability to problems.

> **QUESTIONS AND IDEAS TO THINK ABOUT**
>
> 1. If you have not previously practiced psychodynamic psychotherapy, explore with a patient who is ending their treatment what their feelings about it are. What do they think they have gained from treatment? What concerns might they have about ending treatment? What feelings about the therapist have arisen?
> 2. If you have practiced psychodynamic psychotherapy but not PrFPP, try exploring with a patient who is approaching termination what progress they have made and what concerns they have about ending. Ask the patient to describe what they have learned from the therapy.

WORKSHEET 9.1

Psychodynamic Skills to Address Problems and Their Potential Recurrence

These questions will help you and your therapist summarize progress on problems, consider vulnerabilities to recurrence, and discuss helpful interventions and skills designed to address them.

Are you able to notice when your problems are being triggered? Can you identify the situations and feelings that contribute to this?

Are you able to recognize and work with how your past contributes to your problems?

Are you able to identify how your views and expectations of yourself and others contribute to your problems?

(continued)

From *Skills Training in Psychodynamic Psychotherapy*, by Fredric N. Busch. Copyright © 2026 The Guilford Press. Permission to photocopy this worksheet, or to download and print additional copies (*www.guilford.com/busch-forms*), is granted to purchasers of this book for personal use or use with clients; see copyright page for details.

Psychodynamic Skills to Address Problems (page 2 of 2)

Do you recognize how conflicts about feelings and wishes contribute to your problems?

How have your misunderstandings of others' feelings and expectations contributed to your problems? How do you address these misconceptions?

What behavioral changes have you found helpful in dealing with your problems?

References

Abraham, K. (1911). Notes on the psycho-analytical investigation and treatment of manic depressive insanity and allied conditions. In *Selected papers on psychoanalysis* (pp. 137-156). Hogarth Press.

American Psychiatric Association. (2022). *Diagnostic and statistical manual of mental disorders* (5th ed., text rev.). American Psychiatric Press.

Arlow, J. A. (1963). Conflict, regression, and symptom formation. *International Journal of Psychoanalysis, 44*, 12-22.

Arrindell, W., Emmelkamp, P. M. G., Monsma, A., & Brilman, E. (1983). The role of perceived parental rearing practices in the etiology of phobic disorders: A controlled study. *British Journal of Psychiatry, 143*, 183-187.

Bateman, A., & Fonagy, P. (2016). *Mentalization-based treatment for personality disorders*. Oxford University Press.

Bowlby J (1973). *Attachment and loss, Vol. 2: Attachment, anxiety and anger*. Basic Books.

Bucci, W. (1997). Symptoms and symbols: A multiple code theory of somatization. *Psychoanalytic Inquiry, 17*, 151-172.

Busch, F. N. (Ed.). (2008). *Mentalization: Theoretical considerations, research findings, and clinical implications*. Analytic Press.

Busch, F. N. (2017). A model for integrating actual neurotic or unrepresented states and symbolized aspects of intrapsychic conflict. *Psychoanalytic Quarterly, 85*, 75-108.

Busch, F. N. (2018). *Psychodynamic approaches to behavioral change*. American Psychiatric Press.

Busch, F. N. (2022). *Problem focused psychodynamic psychotherapy*. American Psychiatric Press.

Busch, F. N. (2024). Addressing dissociated representations of self and others in the treatment of posttraumatic syndromes. *American Journal of Psychotherapy, 77*, 95-98.

Busch, F. N., Cooper, A. M., Klerman, G. L., Shapiro, T., & Shear, M. K. (1991). Neurophysiological, cognitive-behavioral and psychoanalytic approaches to panic disorder: Toward an integration. *Psychoanalytic Inquiry, 11*, 316-332.

Busch, F. N., Milrod, B. L., Chen C., & Singer M. (2021). *Trauma focused psychodynamic psychotherapy*. Oxford University Press.

Busch, F. N., Milrod, B. L., Singer, M., & Aronson, A. (2012). *Panic-focused psychodynamic psychotherapy, eXtended range*. Routledge.

Busch, F. N., Rudden, M. G., & Shapiro, T. (2016). *Psychodynamic treatment of depression* (2nd ed.). American Psychiatric Press.

Busch, F. N., Shear, M. K., Cooper, A. M., Shapiro, T., & Leon, A. (1995). An empirical study of defense mechanisms in panic disorder. *Journal of Nervous and Mental Disease, 183*, 299–303.

Cassorla, R. M. (2013). When the analyst becomes stupid: An attempt to understand enactment using Bion's theory of thinking. *Psychoanalytic Quarterly, 82*, 323–360.

Clarkin, J. F., Levy, K. N., Lenzenweger, M. F., & Kernberg, O. F. (2007). Evaluating three treatments for borderline personality disorder: A multiwave study. *American Journal of Psychiatry, 64*(6), 922–928.

Cooper, A. M. (1987). Changes in psychoanalytic ideas: Transference interpretation. *Journal of the American Psychoanalytic Association, 35*(1), 77–98.

Fonagy, P. (2008). The mentalization-focused approach to social development. In F. Busch (Ed.). *Mentalization: Theoretical considerations, research findings, and clinical implications* (pp. 3–56). Analytic Press.

Fonagy, P., & Target, M. (1997). Attachment and reflective function: Their role in self-organization. *Development and Psychopathology, 9*, 679–700.

Freud, A. (1936). *The ego and the mechanisms of defense*. International Universities Press.

Freud, S. (1893–1895). Studies on hysteria. In J. Strachey (Ed. & Trans.), *The standard edition of the complete psychological works of Sigmund Freud* (Vol. 2., pp. 1–181). Hogarth Press.

Freud, S. (1905). Fragment of an analysis of a case of hysteria. In J. Strachey (Ed. & Trans.), *The standard edition of the complete psychological works of Sigmund Freud* (Vol. 7, pp. 3–122). Hogarth Press.

Freud, S. (1914). Repeating, remembering, and working through. In J. Strachey (Ed. & Trans.), *The standard edition of the complete psychological works of Sigmund Freud* (Vol. 12, pp. 147–156). Hogarth Press.

Freud, S. (1917). Mourning and melancholia. In J. Strachey (Ed. & Trans.), *The standard edition of the complete psychological works of Sigmund Freud* (Vol. 14, pp. 239–258). Hogarth Press.

Freud, S. (1920). Beyond the pleasure principle. In J. Strachey (Ed. & Trans.), *The standard edition of the complete psychological works of Sigmund Freud* (Vol. 18, pp. 1–64). Hogarth Press.

Freud, S. (1926). Inhibitions, symptoms and anxiety. In J. Strachey (Ed. & Trans.), *The standard edition of the complete psychological works of Sigmund Freud* (Vol. 20, pp. 75–175). Hogarth Press.

Gabbard, G. O. (1995). Countertransference: The emerging common ground. *International Journal of Psychoanalysis, 76*, 475–485.

Isaacs, S. (1948). The nature and function of phantasy. *International Journal of Psychoanalysis, 29*, 73–97.

Jacobson, E. (1964). *The self and the object world*. International Universities Press.

Jacobson, E. (1971). *Depression: Comparative studies of normal, neurotic and psychotic depressions*. International Universities Press.

Kohut, H. (1971). *The analysis of the self*. International Universities Press.

Milrod, B., Chambless, D. L., Gallop, R., Busch, F. N., Schwalberg, M., McCarthy, K. S., et al.

(2016). Psychotherapies for panic disorder: A tale of two sites. *Journal of Clinical Psychiatry, 77*, 927-935.

Milrod, B., Leon, A. C., Busch, F. N., Rudden, M., Schwalberg, M., Clarkin, J., et al. (2007). A randomized controlled clinical trial of psychoanalytic psychotherapy for panic disorder. *American Journal of Psychiatry, 164*, 265-272.

Mitchell (1988). *Relational concepts in psychoanalysis: An integration.* Harvard University Press.

Parker, G. (1979). Reported parental characteristics of agoraphobics and social phobics. *British Journal of Psychiatry, 135*, 555-560.

Perry, S., Cooper, A. M., & Michels, R. (1987). The psychodynamic formulation: Its purpose, structure, and clinical application. *American Journal of Psychiatry, 144*(5), 543-550.

Sandler, J. (1976). Countertransference and role-responsiveness. *International Review of Psychoanalysis, 3*, 43-47.

Shapiro, T. (1992). The concept of unconscious fantasy. *Journal of Clinical Psychoanalysis, 1*, 517-524.

Shear, M. K., Cooper, A. M., Klerman, G. L., Busch, F. N., & Shapiro, T. (1993). A psychodynamic model of panic disorder. *American Journal of Psychiatry, 150*, 859-866.

Silove, D. (1986). Perceived parental characteristics and reports of early parental deprivation in agoraphobic patients. *Australian and New Zealand Journal of Psychiatry, 20*(3), 365-369.

Slade, A., Sadler, L. S., Eaves, T., & Webb, D. L. (2023). *Enhancing attachment and reflective parenting in clinical practice: A Minding the Baby approach.* Guilford Press.

Stern, D. B. (2015). [Review of] *Unrepresented States and the Construction of Meaning: Clinical and Theoretical Contributions,* ed. H. B. Levine, G. S. Reed & D. Scarfone. *International Journal of Psychoanalysis, 96*, 493-498.

Stone, L. (1973). On resistance to the psychoanalytic process. In B. B. Rubenstein (Ed.), *Psychoanalysis and contemporary science* (Vol. 2, pp. 42-73). Macmillan.

Storebo, O. J., Stoffers-Winterling, J. M., Vollm, B. A., Kongerlev, M. T., Mattivi, J. T., Jorgenson, M. S., et al. (2020). Psychological therapies for people with borderline personality disorder. *Cochrane Database of Systematic Reviews, 5.*

Westen, D., & Gabbard, G. O. (2002). Developments in cognitive neuroscience: II. Implications for theories of transference. *Journal of the American Psychoanalytic Association, 50*(1), 99-134.

Winnicott, D. W. (1965). Ego distortion in terms of true and false self. In *The maturational processes and the facilitating environment* (pp. 140-152). International Universities Press.

Yeomans, F. E., Clarkin, J. F., & Kernberg, O. F. (2015). *Transference-focused psychotherapy for borderline personality disorder: A clinical guide.* American Psychiatric Press.

Index

Note. *f* following a page number indicates a figure

Acting in, 17. *See also* Transference
Acting out, 125, 126. *See also* Defenses/defense mechanisms
Addiction, 38-39, 57-58. *See also* Substance use
Aggression, 13, 15, 186
Aggressive wishes/fantasies
　identifying intrapsychic conflicts and, 110-112, 113-117
　intrapsychic conflicts and, 7, 109
　regression and, 15
　See also Fantasies; Wishes
Agoraphobic symptoms, 59-60
Alcohol use. *See* Substance use
All-or-none thinking, 142-144
Ambivalence, 9. *See also* Defenses/defense mechanisms
Anger
　compromise formation and, 126
　defenses and, 9-10, 120-121, 122-123
　directed towards the self, 121, 122, 126
　identifying behavioral problems, 30-31
　intrapsychic conflicts and, 7, 109-111, 113-117
　mentalization skills and, 140-142
　regression and, 15
　representations of self and others and, 99-100
　transference and, 16-17
　underlying dynamics that contribute to problems and, 40-41
　unsymbolized states and, 10-11
　working-through process and, 174, 176
Angry fantasies, 7. *See also* Fantasies
Anxiety
　conflict/defense theory and, 20-21
　defenses and, 120-121, 122, 124-125
　formulation and, 152-156, 157-166
　identifying symptoms and, 26-28
　intrapsychic conflicts and, 7, 8, 109-110, 119
　linking technique and, 60-64, 63*f*
　mentalization skills and, 12-13, 133-134
　problem identification and, 32-33, 37-38
　readiness for ending treatment and, 195-198, 201-207
　regression and, 15
　relevance of developmental experiences to current problems, 68-74, 70*f*
　return to treatment and, 208-210
　somatic symptoms and, 13-14
　transference and, 17
　working-through process and, 175-177, 181-186, 187-188
　worksheets and handouts for, 45-46
　See also Anxiety disorders
Anxiety disorders
　defenses and, 120-121
　intrapsychic conflicts and, 109
　readiness for ending treatment and, 193-194
　working-through process and, 174
　See also Anxiety
Assertiveness
　identifying intrapsychic conflicts and, 113
　personality problems and, 32
　regression and, 15
　working through process and, 174, 177, 183, 186-187
Assessment
　assessing the impact of PrFPP, 167-168, 172-173
　readiness for ending treatment and, 193-207
　See also Clinical interview; Problem identification
Attachment, 14, 120-121

Attachment relationships, 7
Attitudes, 31-32
Autonomy, 15, 117-118
Avoidance, 14, 32, 187-188, 194
Avoidant personality, 32-33, 37-38, 55. *See also* Personality problems

Behavioral change, 2, 194, 198, 201, 204, 207
Behavioral problems
    identifying, 30-31
    personality problems and, 31-32
    readiness for ending treatment and, 194
    repetition compulsion and, 166-167
    representations of self and others and, 86-89
    self-observation and, 59-60
    underlying dynamics that contribute to problems and, 40-41
    working-through process and, 174-175, 177, 183, 185-186
    worksheets and handouts for, 51-55
    See also Compulsive behavior; Impulsive behaviors; Inhibited behaviors; Problem identification
Black-and-white thinking, 142-144
Bodily states
    identifying symptoms and, 29-30
    meanings and functions of problems and, 40
    overview, 10-11, 13-14
    unsymbolized states and, 10-11
    See also Somatic symptoms
Building a scaffold metaphor, 60. *See also* Self-observation

Case formulation. *See* Formulation
Change, 151-152. *See also* Behavioral change
Childhood experiences. *See* Developmental experiences
Children, dealing with, 138-139
Circumstances
    linking technique and, 62-64, 63f, 65f
    relevance of developmental experiences to current problems, 67-74, 70f
    worksheets and handouts for, 75-84
    See also Contexts
Clinical interview
    identifying symptoms and, 26-30
    presenting problems and, 25-26
    problem identification and, 24
    worksheets and handouts and, 3
    See also Assessment
Cluster C personality disorders. *See* Personality disorders
Compromise formation
    conflict/defense theory and, 20-21
    defense mechanisms and, 10
    overview, 10, 126-127
Compulsive behavior
    problem identification and, 25-26
    readiness for ending treatment and, 198-201
    repetition compulsion and, 166-167
    working-through process and, 179-181

    worksheets and handouts for, 192
    See also Behavioral problems; Impulsive behaviors
Conflict/defense theory, 19, 20-21. *See also* Compromise formation; Conflicts; Defenses/defense mechanisms; Intrapsychic conflicts
Conflicts
    formulation and, 153, 154-155, 156, 157-158, 163, 165
    readiness for ending treatment and, 194, 198, 200, 203, 207
    working-through process and, 174-175, 176, 180, 182, 185
    See also Intrapsychic conflicts
Conflicts with others, 136, 146-147, 194. *See also* Interpersonal problems; Relationship problems
Contexts
    formulation and, 152-153, 154, 155, 158, 159, 160-161, 162-165
    overview, 2
    readiness for ending treatment and, 194
    working-through process and, 174-175, 180, 182, 185
    See also Circumstances; Triggers
Control, loss of, 123
Core problems, 23. *See also* Problem identification
Core wishes, 7. *See also* Wishes
Countertransference, 17-18, 21-22. *See also* Therapeutic relationship
Cultural factors, 40, 69

Defenses/defense mechanisms
    conflict/defense theory and, 20-21
    denial and, 38-39
    formulation and, 151, 153, 154-155, 156, 158, 163-165
    intrapsychic conflicts and, 7
    overview, 8-10, 109-110, 120-126
    representations of self and others and, 98
    self-observation and, 59-60
    working-through process and, 174-175, 176, 180, 182, 185
    worksheets and handouts for, 128-129
Denial
    overview, 9-10, 121, 125
    problem identification and, 36, 38-39
    working-through process and, 176
    See also Defenses/defense mechanisms
Dependency
    identifying intrapsychic conflicts and, 111, 115-118
    intrapsychic conflicts and, 7
    regression and, 15-16
    working-through process and, 174
Dependent wishes, 110. *See also* Wishes
Depression
    defenses and, 122, 124-125
    formulation and, 152-157, 158-162
    identifying symptoms and, 28-29
    intrapsychic conflicts and, 7, 109
    linking technique and, 60-64, 63f

Depression (continued)
  mentalization skills and, 133–134, 140–144
  problem identification and, 28–29, 33–34
  readiness for ending treatment and, 204–207
  regression and, 15–16
  relevance of developmental experiences to current problems, 68–71, 70f
  representations of self and others and, 86–89
  symptoms and, 13
  transference and, 17
  working-through process and, 177–179, 183–186
  worksheets and handouts for, 47–48
Depressive disorders, 7, 15. *See also* Depression
Devaluation, 121, 125. *See also* Defenses/defense mechanisms
Developmental experiences
  formulation and, 101, 102, 153, 154, 158, 159, 161–162
  intrapsychic conflicts and, 6–7
  linking technique and, 62–64, 63f, 65f, 93–95
  mentalization skills and, 136–138
  overview, 2
  readiness for ending treatment and, 194, 197, 200, 203, 206
  regression and, 15–16
  relevance of to current problems, 67–74, 70f
  repetition compulsion and, 166–167
  working-through process and, 174–175, 176, 180, 185
  worksheets and handouts for, 82–84, 107–108
Diary
  formulation and, 161–162
  linking technique and, 60–64, 63f, 65f
  monitoring thoughts, feelings, and reactions surrounding problems, 60–64, 63f, 65f
  relevance of developmental experiences to current problems, 67–74, 70f
  using to address impulsive behaviors and inhibitions, 65–67
  See also Self-observation; Worksheets and handouts
Dissociated states
  overview, 123
  relational/interpersonal model and, 21–22
  representations of self and others and, 99–100
  symbolization models and, 19
  See also Defenses/defense mechanisms
Drug use. *See* Substance use
Dynamic unconscious, 6. *See also* Unconscious

Early experiences. *See* Developmental experiences
Early relationships, 11. *See also* Relationship problems
Emotions
  formulation and, 152–153, 154, 155, 158, 159, 160–161, 162, 163–165
  readiness for ending treatment and, 194
  self-reflective skills and, 23–24
  transference and, 16–17
  working-through process and, 174–175
  See also Feelings
Enactments, 18–19, 21–22, 67

Ending treatment. *See* Termination
Environmental factors, 19
Evaluation. *See* Assessment; Clinical interview
Expectations
  mentalization skills and, 144–145
  readiness for ending treatment and, 198, 201, 203, 206, 207
  representations of self and others and, 20
  working-through process and, 181–182
Experiences, developmental. *See* Developmental experiences

Fantasies
  conflict/defense theory and, 20–21
  defenses and, 120–121
  intrapsychic conflicts and, 6–7, 109–120
  overview, 2
  readiness for ending treatment and, 194
  unsymbolized states and, 10–11
  worksheets and handouts for, 128–132
  See also Wishes
Feelings
  identifying intrapsychic conflicts and, 110–112
  intrapsychic conflicts and, 6–7
  linking technique and, 62–64, 63f, 65f
  monitoring thoughts, feelings, and reactions surrounding problems, 60–64, 63f, 65f
  problem identification and, 36–38
  readiness for ending treatment and, 194, 198, 200, 203, 206–207
  relevance of developmental experiences to current problems, 67–74, 70f
  repetition compulsion and, 166–167
  self-reflective skills and, 23–24
  unsymbolized states and, 10–11
  worksheets and handouts for, 75–84, 128–132
  See also Emotions
Formulation
  building, 100–103
  conflicts and defenses, 153, 154–155, 156–157, 158–159, 163, 165
  contexts and emotions surrounding problems, 152–153, 154, 155, 158, 159, 160–161, 162, 163–165
  developmental history, 101, 102, 153, 154, 158, 159, 161–162
  interconnection between problems, 166
  interventions based on, 101, 102–103, 155–157, 160–162, 163–166
  mentalization impairments, 153–154, 155, 157, 158, 159, 163, 165
  overview, 148, 151–152
  problem list, 100, 101, 102, 154, 159, 162
  repetition compulsion and, 166–167
  representations of self and others and, 89–90, 100, 101, 102, 153, 154, 156, 158, 159, 161–162, 165
  transference and, 157
  working-through process and, 174–175
  worksheets and handouts for, 170–173

Goals, 174–175
Guided interviews. *See* Clinical interview
Guilt
   conflict/defense theory and, 20–21
   intrapsychic conflicts and, 7, 109–110, 119
   mentalization skills and, 136–138, 140–142
   problem identification and, 36–39
   underlying dynamics that contribute to problems and, 40–41
   working-through process and, 186

Handouts. *See* Worksheets and handouts
Home practice. *See* Worksheets and handouts
Humor, 120, 126. *See also* Defenses/defense mechanisms

Idealization, 121, 122, 125. *See also* Defenses/defense mechanisms
Identification of problems. *See* Problem identification
Identification with the aggressor, 125. *See also* Defenses/defense mechanisms
Impulses, 19, 32. *See also* Impulsive behaviors
Impulsive behaviors
   barriers to recognizing problems and, 36
   identifying, 30–31
   linking technique and, 64, 65*f*
   readiness for ending treatment and, 198–201
   self-observation and, 59
   splitting and, 123–125
   working-through process and, 179–181
   worksheets and handouts for, 53–54, 65–67, 78–79, 192
   See also Behavioral problems; Compulsive behavior
Inhibited behaviors
   identifying behavioral problems, 30–31
   self-observation and, 59
   using diaries and worksheets to address, 65–67
   worksheets and handouts for, 51–52, 80–81
   See also Behavioral problems
Internal representations, 11–12. *See also* Representations of self and others
Interpersonal problems
   conflicts with others, 136, 146–147, 194
   formulation and, 162–166
   intrapsychic conflicts and, 7–8
   mentalization skills and, 12–13, 140–148
   overview, 21–22
   readiness for ending treatment and, 194, 195–201
   working-through process and, 181–186
   See also Conflicts with others; Relationship problems
Interventions
   formulation and, 101, 102–103, 155–157, 160–162, 163–166
   intrapsychic conflicts and, 112
   See also Mentalization skills
Interview, clinical. *See* Clinical interview
Intrapsychic conflicts
   building a formulation and, 103
   identifying, 110–120
   intrapsychic conflicts and, 8
   overview, 6–7, 109–110
   readiness for ending treatment and, 194
   regression and, 15
   relevance of developmental experiences to current problems, 67–74, 70*f*
   representations of self and others and, 98
   self-observation and, 59–60
   transference and, 16–17
   worksheets and handouts for, 128–129
   See also Conflicts
Intrapsychic factors, 6–13
Intrusion, 11

Language, 5–6, 24
Linking technique, 62–64, 63*f*, 65*f*, 91–95
Loss, 15, 17
Loss of control, 123

Manualization of treatment, 1
Marital conflict, 146–147. *See also* Relationship problems
Mental representations. *See* Representations of self and others
Mentalization skills
   in dealing with children, 138–139
   expanding the use of, 147–148
   formulation and, 153–154, 155, 157, 158, 159, 163, 165–166
   overview, 2, 12–13, 127, 133–138
   readiness for ending treatment and, 194
   relationship problems and, 144–147
   self-criticism and, 139–144
   self-esteem and, 139–140
   working-through process and, 174–175, 177, 180, 182, 183, 185
   worksheets and handouts for, 149–150
Metacommunication, 21–22
Motivation, 13, 15–16, 23–24

Narcissistic personality problems, 33–34. *See also* Personality problems
Numbing, 123. *See also* Defenses/defense mechanisms; Dissociated states

Object relations theory, 19, 20
Obsessive–compulsive disorder, 142–144
Other representations. *See* Representations of self and others
Overburdened feelings
   readiness for ending treatment and, 195–198, 204–207
   working-through process and, 177–179

Panic disorder, 7, 11–12. *See also* Panic/panic attacks
Panic/panic attacks
   defense mechanisms and, 10
   defenses and, 120–121, 122–123
   identifying intrapsychic conflicts and, 115, 116–117

Panic/panic attacks *(continued)*
  intrapsychic conflicts and, 7, 8
  linking technique and, 62–64, 63f
  readiness for ending treatment and, 201–204
  regression and, 15
  relevance of developmental experiences to current problems, 68–74, 70f
  representations of self and others and, 11–12
  somatic symptoms and, 13–14
  working-through process and, 174, 175–177, 181–183
  worksheets and handouts for, 77
Passive aggression, 120–121, 122, 125, 187–188. *See also* Defenses/defense mechanisms
Personality disorders, 7, 32–34, 109. *See also* Personality problems
Personality problems, 31–34, 36, 40–41. *See also* Personality disorders; Problem identification
Prediction, 20
Presenting problems, 24–26. *See also* Problem identification; Problem list
Problem identification
  barriers to recognizing problems, 35–36
  behavioral problems, 30–31
  building a formulation and, 100, 101, 102
  cultural factors and, 40
  denial and, 38–39
  guilt or shame and, 36–38
  identifying intrapsychic conflicts and, 110–120
  interconnection between problems, 166
  linking representations of self and others to, 91–93
  meanings and functions of problems and, 39–40
  overview, 23, 24–39
  personality problems, 31–34
  presenting problems, 24–26
  relationship problems, 34–35
  self-observation and, 59–60
  self-reflective skills and, 23–24
  symptoms, 26–30
  underlying dynamics that contribute to problems, 40–41
  worksheets and handouts for, 42–58, 170–173
  See also Behavioral problems; Personality problems; Problem list; Relationship problems; Self-observation; Symptoms
Problem list
  construction of, 23, 39, 40
  formulation and, 100, 101, 102, 151, 154, 159, 162
  overview, 24, 32
  readiness for ending treatment and, 197, 202, 205–206
  See also Problem identification
Problem-focused psychodynamic psychotherapy (PrFPP)
  assessing the impact of, 167–169, 172–173
  formulation and, 100–103
  overview, 1–2, 5–6, 23, 24, 42
  return to treatment and, 207–210
Problems, working through. *See* Working-through process

Prohibitions, internalized, 6–7
Projection, 109–110, 121, 122. *See also* Defenses/defense mechanisms
Psychoanalytic models of the mind, 19–22
Psychodynamic concepts, 5–6
Psychodynamic formulation. *See* Formulation
Psychodynamic skills
  overview, 2, 194
  readiness for ending treatment and, 197–198, 203–204, 206–207
Psychoeducation, 2
Psychotherapeutic interventions. *See* Interventions

Reaction formation, 9–10, 120, 121, 122, 125. *See also* Defenses/defense mechanisms
Reactions
  monitoring thoughts, feelings, and reactions surrounding problems, 60–64, 63f, 65f
  relevance of developmental experiences to current problems, 67–74, 70f
  worksheets and handouts for, 75–84
Recurrence of problems
  return to treatment and, 207–210
  working-through process and, 174–175, 211–212
Regression, 15–16
Regressive defense, 20–21. *See also* Defenses/defense mechanisms
Rejection
  intrapsychic conflicts and, 109–110
  mentalization skills and, 144–145
  object relations theory and, 20
  representations of self and others and, 11, 90, 95–98
Relational/interpersonal model, 19, 21–22
Relationship problems
  barriers to recognizing problems and, 36
  conflicts with others, 136, 146–147, 194
  defenses and, 124–125
  identifying, 34–35
  identifying intrapsychic conflicts and, 111–112
  mentalization skills and, 135–136, 144–147
  relational/interpersonal model and, 21–22
  representations of self and others and, 11
  underlying dynamics that contribute to problems and, 40–41
  worksheets and handouts for, 56
  See also Conflicts with others; Interpersonal problems; Problem identification
Repetition compulsion, 166–167
Representations of self and others
  building a formulation and, 100, 101, 102
  challenging, 96–98
  developing thoughts to counter, 98–99
  dissociated self and other representations, 99–100
  feeling trapped, 95–96
  formulating, 89–90
  formulation and, 153, 154, 156, 158, 159, 161–162, 165
  identifying, 91

linking technique and, 62–64, 63f, 65f, 91–95
  mentalization and, 127
  object relations theory and, 20
  overview, 2, 11–12, 85–89
  readiness for ending treatment and, 194, 198, 200, 203–204, 206–207
  relational/interpersonal model and, 21–22
  relevance of developmental experiences to current problems, 67–74, 70f
  symbolization models and, 19
  viewing oneself as a failure, 95
  working-through process and, 174–175, 176, 180, 181–182, 185, 187
  worksheets and handouts for, 104–108
Repression, 121, 125. See also Defenses/defense mechanisms
Resistance, 14–15
Reviewing a video metaphor, 60. See also Self-observation

Self representations. See Representations of self and others
Self-criticism
  formulation and, 152–157
  intrapsychic conflicts and, 7
  mentalization skills and, 134, 139–144
  object relations theory and, 20
  regression and, 15–16
  representations of self and others and, 86–89
  symptoms and, 13
  working-through process and, 177–179, 186–187
Self-directed anger, 121, 122, 126. See also Anger; Defenses/defense mechanisms
Self-esteem
  defenses and, 121
  mentalization skills and, 134, 139–140, 148
  return to treatment and, 208–210
Self-observation
  monitoring thoughts, feelings, and reactions surrounding problems, 60–64, 63f, 65f
  overview, 2, 59–60
  working-through process and, 177
  See also Diary; Problem identification
Self-punishment, 7, 109
Self-reflective skills, 23–24
Self-views
  challenging, 96–99
  mentalization skills and, 139–144
  readiness for ending treatment and, 194, 198, 200, 203, 206
  representations of self and others and, 11, 95
  working-through process and, 181–182
Self-worth, 183–186
Separation
  fear of, 9
  identifying intrapsychic conflicts and, 111, 115–118
  regression and, 15
  transference and, 17

Sexual fantasies/wishes
  identifying intrapsychic conflicts and, 113, 119–120
  intrapsychic conflicts and, 7, 109–110
  See also Fantasies; Wishes
Sexual feelings, 113
Shame, 20–21, 36–38
Skills, psychodynamic, 2, 194
Somatic symptoms
  identifying, 29–30
  meanings and functions of problems and, 40
  overview, 13–14, 19
  worksheets and handouts for, 49–50
  See also Bodily states; Symptoms
Somatization, 9, 20–21, 122–123, 125–126. See also Defenses/defense mechanisms
Splitting, 123–125, 187. See also Defenses/defense mechanisms
"Staging area," 59–60
Substance use
  formulation and, 162–166
  problem identification and, 36, 38–39
  readiness for ending treatment and, 195–198
  worksheets and handouts for, 57–58
Suppression, 120, 126. See also Defenses/defense mechanisms
Symbolization, 13, 19, 20–21
Symptoms
  identifying, 26–30
  intrapsychic conflicts and, 109–110
  overview, 13–14
  relevance of developmental experiences to current problems, 67–74, 70f
  return to treatment and, 207–210
  self-observation and, 59–60
  underlying dynamics that contribute to problems and, 40–41
  using diaries and worksheets to address, 65–67
  working-through process and, 174–175
  See also Behavioral problems; Problem identification; Somatic symptoms

Termination
  assessing the readiness for, 193–207
  overview, 2, 189, 193
  return to treatment and, 207–210
  working-through process and, 211–212
Therapeutic relationship, 16–17, 21–22. See also Transference
Thoughts
  linking technique and, 62–64, 63f, 65f
  monitoring thoughts, feelings, and reactions surrounding problems, 60–64, 63f, 65f
  relevance of developmental experiences to current problems, 67–74, 70f
  repetition compulsion and, 166–167
  representations of self and others and, 98–99
  self-reflective skills and, 23–24
  worksheets and handouts for, 75–84

Transference
    conflict/defense theory and, 20–21
    formulation and, 157, 165
    overview, 1, 16–17
    relational/interpersonal model and, 21–22
    termination and, 196, 199
    working-through process and, 177, 180, 183, 185
Trapped feelings, 95–96, 177–179
Trauma
    intrapsychic conflicts and, 6–7
    repetition compulsion and, 166–167
    representations of self and others and, 86–89, 99
Triggers
    overview, 2, 3
    readiness for ending treatment and, 197, 200, 203, 206
    working-through process and, 176, 180, 182, 185
    See also Contexts

Unconscious
    conflict/defense theory and, 20–21
    meanings and functions of problems and, 40
    resistance and, 14
    role of in symptoms and problems, 6–8
    splitting and, 123
    See also Intrapsychic conflicts
Undoing, 9–10, 120, 125. *See also* Defenses/defense mechanisms
Unsymbolized states, 10–11

Whirlpool metaphor, 60. *See also* Self-observation
Wishes
    conflict/defense theory and, 20–21
    intrapsychic conflicts and, 6–7, 109–110
    readiness for ending treatment and, 198, 200, 203, 207
    worksheets and handouts for, 128–132
    See also Fantasies
Working-through process
    avoidance, 187–188
    compulsive behavior, 179–181
    overburdened feelings, 177–179
    overview, 174–188
    panic, 175–177, 181–183
    self-criticism and, 186–187
    self-worth, 183–186
    worksheets and handouts for, 190–192
Worksheets and handouts
    Handout 2.1: Introduction to the Treatment, 24, 42
    Handout 3.1: Paying Attention to Circumstances, Thoughts, Feelings, and Reactions Associated with Problems, 60, 75
    how to use, 2–3, 24
    overview, 2, 5
    using to address impulsive behaviors and inhibitions, 65–67

Worksheet 2.1: Initial Identification or Problems, 25, 33–34, 43–44
Worksheet 2.2: Initial Evaluation of Anxiety, 26–30, 45–46
Worksheet 2.3: Initial Evaluation of Depression, 28–29, 47–48
Worksheet 2.4: Initial Evaluation of Somatic Symptoms, 29–30, 49–50
Worksheet 2.5: Initial Evaluation of Inhibited Behaviors, 30–31, 51–52
Worksheet 2.6: Initial Evaluation of Behaviors That Are Difficult to Control, 30–31, 53–54
Worksheet 2.7: Initial Evaluation of Avoidant Tendencies, 32–33, 55
Worksheet 2.8: Initial Evaluation of Relationship Problems, 35, 56
Worksheet 2.9: Initial Evaluation of Addiction Problems, 38–39, 57–58
Worksheet 3.1: Monitoring Circumstances, Thoughts, Feelings and Reactions Surrounding Problems, 3, 60–64, 63f, 65f, 76, 162
Worksheet 3.2: Assessing Triggers and Content of Panic Attacks, 63–64, 77
Worksheet 3.3: Exploring Not Acting on Impulsive Behavior, 65–67, 78–79, 164
Worksheet 3.4: Exploring Enacting an Inhibited Behavior, 67, 72, 80–81
Worksheet 3.5: Exploring Developmental History, 67–74, 70f, 82–84
Worksheet 4.1: Self and Other Representations: How You See and What You Expect from Yourself and Others, 86–89, 104–106
Worksheet 4.2: Linking Self and Other Representations to Early Experiences: Consider How You Felt with Your Caregivers When You Were Growing Up, 94–95, 107–108
Worksheet 5.1: Conflicts about Feelings and Fantasies, 110–112, 128–129
Worksheet 5.2: How You Manage Your Feelings and Wishes, 125, 130–132
Worksheet 6.1: Understanding What Is Happening in Your Own and Others' Minds, 134–136, 149–150
Worksheet 7.1: Identifying Contributors to Your Problems, 151, 154, 162, 170–171
Worksheet 7.2: Assessing the Impact of Treatment, 152, 167, 172–173
Worksheet 8.1: Elements of Working Through Problems, 175, 176, 190–191
Worksheet 8.2: Holding Back on Impulsive Behaviors, 181, 192
Worksheet 9.1: Psychodynamic Skills to Address Problems and Their Potential Recurrence, 194, 197–198, 200–201, 203–204, 206–207, 211–212